The Art and Etiquette of Polyamory

The Art and Etiquette of Polyamory

A HANDS-ON GUIDE TO OPEN SEXUAL RELATIONSHIPS

Françoise Simpère
Translation by Joanna Oseman

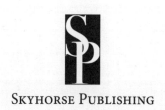

SKYHORSE PUBLISHING

Skyhorse Publishing books may be purchased in bulk at special
discounts for sales promotion, corporate gifts, fund-raising, or
educational purposes. Special editions can also be created to
specifications. For details, contact the Special Sales Department,
Skyhorse Publishing, 307 West 36th Street, 11th Floor, New
York, NY 10018 or info@skyhorsepublishing.com.

www.skyhorsepublishing.com

10 9 8 7 6 5 4 3 2 1

Library of Congress Cataloging-in-Publication Data

Simpère, Françoise.
 The art and etiquette of polyamory : a hands-on guide to open
sexual relationships / Françoise Simpère.
     p. cm.
 Includes bibliographical references.
 ISBN 978-1-61608-193-5 (pbk. : alk. paper)
 1. Non-monogamous relationships. 2. Sexual ethics. I. Title.
 HQ980.S56 2011
 306.84'23–dc22

                         2010050918
 Printed in Canada

FRANÇOISE SIMPÈRE

Françoise Simpère is a journalist, writer, and author of, among others, *Aimer plusieurs hommes* (*To Love Several Men*), *L'algue fatale* (*The Deadly Seaweed*), *Des désirs et des hommes* (*Men and Desire*), *Bien dans l'eau,bien dans sa peau* (*Feeling Good in Water . . . and in Yourself*), *Les latitudes amoureuses* (*Latitudes of Love*), *Ce qui trouble Lola* (*The Trouble With Lola*), *Il n'est jamais trop tard pour aimer plusieurs hommes* (*It's Never Too Late To Love More Than One Man*), and *Le bonheur est un art subtil* (*The Subtle Art of Happiness*). Her areas of interest, present in all of her works, are eroticism, environmentalism, and social issues. As the director of the Senso collection (from French publishing house Editions Blanche), she writes fiction for television and the big screen and is also a documentary contributor. She was the subject of the documentary *La grande amoureuse*, directed by the Québécois

Martine Asselin, which has aired several times in Québec since its production in 2007. A freelance journalist, she also regularly updates her blog Jouer au monde *http://fsimpere.over-blog.com.*

For my daughters, Anne-Sophie and Lauranne,

May their love lives be the most beautiful in the world.

Contents

"Love is sharing everything you wish to share with another, and to live the rest as you see fit. This is the only kind of love that can last."

—Benoîte Groult, May 2008

"The boundary between love and friendship has been covered in barbwire . . . but love and friendship share the same innocence, between love and friendship, then, what is the difference."

—Henri Tachan

"I hope for nothing, I fear nothing, I am free."

—Nikos Kazantzakis, Cretan poet imprisoned for twelve years

The Art and Etiquette of Polyamory

Foreword

To she who changed my life . . .

Dear Françoise,
    We don't know each other, yet I already feel like I know so much about you. Three years ago, you were responsible (albeit unintentionally) for saving my relationship. My wife and I were going through a divorce at the time and I had met a woman through an internet forum. I was at a point where I couldn't see what there was left to hope for from my relationship with my partner, with whom I have a wonderful little boy. Then one day, wandering the aisles of Fnac,[1] I came across your

---

1 Translator's note: Fnac is an international entertainment retail chain, the largest of its kind in France.

book, *It's Never Too Late To Love More Than One Man.*[2] Why I was drawn to this book among the thousands on display I'll never know, but I quickly read the blurb and bought it immediately. That very night I picked it up and could not tear myself away! I read it and turned straight around and read it again.

Words of truth can light up the world for some people, and, at that instant, your truth became mine. My wife and I had been seeing each other again over the previous few months. We were living apart but were getting on well again, better and better as time went on, and the divorce was beginning to seem like a ridiculous idea. My first wife had also left me because I had been unfaithful, and I was beginning to wonder, "Am I going to get divorced every seven years, just because I'm interested in other women?"

I mentioned your book to my "future ex" and asked her if she would read it. "What she says here is what I am saying to you; what she feels, I feel," I told her. For months, years even, I had been searching for a way to express my discontent and to articulate my broad feelings about love and friendship between men and women.

Since then, my wife and I have rediscovered each other, bought another house together, and are expecting a baby in July. Before the child was conceived, we spent a long time deciding whether we really wanted to live "this way" in the years to come. Last year my wife met a man with whom she had a relationship that lasted a few months. I had never seen her so radiant, nor had

---

2 Ed. La Martinière 2002, Pocket 2004.

she ever shown me as much affection and tenderness as at that time. Eventually she broke it off with this man because he could not understand our situation and wanted her to leave me for him. He would not give up, and so she quietly slipped away.

Hardly anybody around us is fully able to understand our lifestyle, without even mentioning our families, to whom it would be impossible to explain just half of what I have written to you. I am certainly still the driving force behind this lifestyle change. My wife is generally comfortable with the situation, but on any given day jealousy can take her for an unexpected spin. I do my best to help her, to reassure her of my love.

I have been thinking of writing this to you for a long time now, but I told myself that you had bigger fish to fry and that my testimonial would be useless. But then I saw you on the Mireille Dumas television show and the idea reared its head again. Not that the wondrous forces of coincidence didn't play their role in this too: You recently left a comment on the blog of a friend of mine who is as big a fan of yours as I am. I took the opportunity to copy down the mailing address you posted and to finally send you the letter which has been so close to my heart. I hope that one day I will have the honor of meeting you . . . "

I contacted this gentleman, V, who asked if I would be his child's godmother—"Without you, he wouldn't be here." A few months later I met V, his partner, and the baby. We kept in contact and even spent a weekend in the country with other readers for whom my book and blog[3] had been the helping hand into a new kind of love life, or, for some, had provided comfort in the knowledge that they were not alone in their choice to live a lifestyle that embraces romantic diversity.

This letter and dozens like it, along with all of the emails, phone calls, and meeting requests that I received, confirmed that *To Love Several Men* had touched on a sensitive area. Of all my books, this was the one that earned me the most interviews and invitations on both radio and television—to the point that I sometimes have to remind people that romantic plurality is not my only interest, and that there are many other subjects about which I would like to be interviewed.

Through the travels I embark upon in my work as a scientific journalist, I often meet researchers, politicians, and sociologists. And there have been many times when, at the end of a meeting, these people approach me about a television program they saw me on and spontaneously bombard me with their marital problems and fantasies!

Chance brought me the secret diary of an elderly lady who has now passed away. In the pages, written during the war, she speaks of her husband, who encouraged her to have lovers while he was away on the front line, "because he couldn't bear the thought of his dear wife withering away and hoped to find her as impassioned as ever when he returned on leave." And so it was. The couple continued their romantic escapades well after the war had ended—escapades which kept the fire of love and beauty burning, if the passionate glances she still shot to her elderly husband and the pure radiance

---

3 Jouer au monde, *http://fsimpere.over-blog.com.*

of this eighty-year-old lady, glowing with *joie de vivre*, are anything to go by.

Over the years I have ready many books about relationships, a topic which carries as much theoretical baggage as that of psychology, medicine, or sexology. Authors, therefore, are often led to draw radically different conclusions, providing us with the proof that absolute truth in this matter does not exist. Through reading novels and works of sociology, biology, and spirituality, I have been able to better articulate where I stand on the issue of dependence and free will,[4] but my own experiences and those of my correspondents have taught me more than I have learned from any other venue. I receive such extraordinary testimonials from polyamorous men and women, through which they either describe their personal stories or seek my advice, and every one of them is unique. Open relationships, as is their nature, do not conform to any particular model. They are lived in a manner dictated by the personality of each individual or couple, who must constantly reinvent the rules of the game whose very goal is evolution, and not stagnation. While monogamy may forbid having more than one partner in your life, that does not mean that by embracing polyamory you are forced to have multiple partners; it is perfectly possible to be in a phase either of multiple relationships, of a single monogamous one, or perhaps none at all, dependant on desire, which is not linear or fixed in time, but cyclical and constantly changing. I have been touched by the kindness exhibited by the men and women who write to me for advice when

---

4 See Bibliography, pg. 215.

their partner falls in love with somebody else: "I love him/her, I want him/her to be happy, but I don't want to lose what we've built together. How can we reconcile our love with that that he/she has for this other person?" How far we are in this instance from possessiveness and illicit urges . . .

These polyamorous relationships are not the same thing as the "open" relationships popular in the 1970s, or today's trend of swinging, which is extremely rigid in structure.[5] "Polyamory," as it is referred to throughout this book, should be understood to encompass many aspects of freedom, as we will see, and not just those of a sexual and romantic nature, as can sometimes be the case in some polyamorous communities.[6] To embrace this way of life, a complete reprogramming of the "romantic central nervous system," as it were, is necessary. If confronted with the concept without warning or adequate reflection as to its implications, many couples

5 See the chapter "Elsewhere."

6 Translator's note: The author, in wanting to make clear that the form of polyamory to which she refers encompasses many forms of freedom and not merely those of a sexual nature, decided to make this distinction through the coining of a new phrase. The resulting word, "lutinage," is derived from the French verb *lutiner* (to woo/court, to arouse the desire of a woman) and also has connotations of charm and cheerfulness. Those that partake in "lutinage" become "lutins" (masculine) and "lutines" (feminine) in the original French text, terms that conjure up images of mischievous, spritely elves from a parallel universe. However, this term is considered to be almost synonymous with "polyamory" (see www.polyamour. info). For the purpose of this English edition, and for lack of an equivalent term in English, this second term will remain.

could be destroyed by the lifestyle—not because it is a harmful concept in and of itself, but because for them it would be artificial. Las Vegas, the luxury city in the middle of a desert, is an artificial universe that sucks dry the banks of the Colorado River. A possessive man using polyamory as an opportunity to commit adultery would be artificial in this same way. A life of harmony cannot exist without intellectual coherence. One female correspondent wrote, "Poly women yearn for discovery and knowledge, and have devoted a lot of time to pondering the question of freedom. Like the witches of yesteryear, their capacity to think and live in a way that defies the rules of normality is met with a mixture of fascination and hostility. Fortunately, though, this is not the Middle Ages, and it is time to stop burning witches."

I have enjoyed seven years of such conversations with dozens of readers, some of whom have become great friends. Thanks to this, and in part to my own personal development, I have reached the conclusion that polyamory is an individual choice before it is that of the couple, and that it largely surpasses the issue of sexuality. The majority of issues that arise when one loves more than one person do concern the unit of the couple, for the simple reason that single poly men and women, given that they have no official ties, are free to conduct their relationships as they see fit. This does not, of course, exempt them from the obligation that they show respect and consideration to their partners. The required reprogramming of the "romantic central nervous system" and the existential questions raised by polyamory are concerns for both singles and couples.

Polyamory is a global life choice, but its daily application changes on a case-by-case basis. "Think globally, act locally"—this environmentalist slogan fits our topic perfectly, and we will see later that this is by no means a coincidence.

This book is not intended to be a user's manual, but rather a guide that each reader can adapt to his or her own personal life. The following topics will be discussed:

From "Elsewhere" to "Sex": A glossary of the theoretical aspects of polyamory. Each section will be followed by questions that people have asked me over the years, or that I have asked myself at times when no one else could advise me.

Dos and Don'ts: Based on real-life situations, this know-how is by no means all-encompassing, but offers advice for poly men and women as they confront issues for the first time in the midst of a staunchly monogamous world.

Testimonials: These real-life accounts from poly men and women demonstrate the variety of experiences that stem from this principle concept and show the extent to which our patterns of romantic behavior are changing. These testimonials show some of the difficulties encountered as a result of this lifestyle alongside stories of the happiness that it can bring. I am grateful for the trust that these men and women have displayed in agreeing that their words be reproduced here.[7]

---

7 Anonymity was respected where requested.

Definitions

Polyamorous relationships: Simultaneous relationships of a sexual, intellectual, or emotional nature, or a combination of these elements.

Lover: A person with whom one has a relationship outside of the couple. The nature of this relationship may vary.

Partner: A person with whom one shares his or her life. This term is broader than husband/wife, given that many couples are not married but are still life partners, even if they do not live under the same roof.

Poly men/women: Men and women who have polyamorous relationships.

Polyamory: The lifestyle of poly men and women.

Monogamy: The dominant model for life as a couple, understood here to be defined as exclusive monogamy, whereby outside relationships are forbidden.

Every issue raised here may be applied to both sexes. Polyamory's principal characteristic is to practice gender equality while allowing men and women to embrace their individual needs and sensibilities.

Polyamory, as it is presented here, is the result of thirty-five years of life, reflections, and relationship observation. It should go without saying that this does not apply to every single poly man or woman, but is rather an ideal.

WHAT POLYAMORY IS ... AND IS NOT

Elsewhere

Moral rules are not universal—a little travel will show anybody that—nor are they something an individual is born with. Rather, they are the product of historical circumstance or society models. Take, for example, the Mormon Church, for whose members polygamy was practiced during a period when they were subject to much persecution. At that time, many men died in combat, leaving behind wives and children who were destitute and had nowhere to turn. There was no choice but to allow men to marry multiple times, in order that these widows could benefit from the support of a family structure.

Monogamy in the West is justified by the official stance that it is impossible to love more than one person at a time—a dogma that is built upon the confusion of love and passion. In other words, passionate love is an intense, narcissistic feeling of attachment that can simply not be shared. However, it is universally agreed that after its initially passionate stage, love must evolve into the building of a life together in order to stay alive, and this being the case, it is as unreasonable to continue to demand exclusivity as it would be to demand exclusive love for a child or a friend.

The foundations of monogamy can be found at the root of the social values that it reflects. In a society built upon the notion of accumulating goods, it has always been important for men to be able to pass down such goods to any children they may father. Monogamy was something that could guarantee to any given man that the children carried by his partner were indeed his. Today, however, contraception and the ability to prove paternity through DNA testing have rendered this objective unnecessary. Furthermore, the protection offered by monogamy is not infallible: Many husbands have unknowingly raised children who were not their own, just as others have fathered children in adultery, something that meant, at a certain time, that these children could stake no claims on inheritance. The cracks in the walls of the monogamy agreement are a clear sign that, since the rules have been broken from the beginning of time, such a demand of exclusivity is not necessarily the natural thing it was once believed to be.[8]

We must, then, look elsewhere in order to understand why monogamy continues to be the sole accept-

---

8 Take Joseph, for example: husband of Mary but not the father of Jesus Christ.

able model for romantic life.[9] One theory is that monogamy helps to keep couples in a state of latent sexual
frustration, given that they are, on principal, forbidden
to fulfill the desires that confront them in their everyday
lives. In order to quell frustrations, a little compensation
is required: Extensive marketing surveys have shown
that the majority of sales of non-vital goods to individuals are driven by the need for self-affirmation and for the
stimulation of the libido ("He's got the money, he's got
the car, he'll get the girl"—this advertising slogan, like
countless others, shows that marketing exploits sexual
desire in the name of sales). Some studies have even
found a direct correlation between the length of the
blade chosen when purchasing a chainsaw . . . and buy-
er's dreams of virility! Monogamy, therefore, favors con-
sumerism, presented as the key to growth, prosperity,
and, by consequence, happiness within a materialistic
society. One final theory, clearly linked to the previous
one, is that monogamy corresponds directly to values of
ownership and power, as promoted by a market society.
To be married is to be the sole keeper of another being
for one's exclusive enjoyment, much to the satisfaction
of the dominant narcissist who lies dormant in so many
individuals.

This model, however, must be flawed, given that one
in three marriages (one in two in the Paris region) ends
in divorce, not counting the couples who remain married despite a lack of happiness and fulfillment. Logic

9 For those who are happy within the structure of monogamy,
of course, and who do not experience outside desires, there is
no reason to change.

dictates, therefore, that while we may keep this model for the third of households for whom it rings true, we are in need of other romantic options to act not as Band-Aids for the existing one, but rather as new concepts. Unfortunately, it can be extremely difficult to change the logic of thought. We prefer to live with hidden affairs or to look for erotic distractions, but certainly not to question the underlying logic of this model and not to ask ourselves whether another way of thinking is possible.

This intellectual laziness can be found on both the political and economical level: Consider the example of Alan Greenspan, ex-director of the Federal Reserve, who admitted, after twenty years of blind faith in a system of market self-regulation, that "there is a flaw in the system and it must be changed"—many of those would rather try to fix it, shielding their eyes from the glaring fact that the same logic will sooner or later simply reproduce the same level of destruction. The ability of the liberal financial system to end poverty is widely contradicted, but many economists continue, with unbelievable mental stubbornness, to support the notion that this poverty is accidental and refuse to look to a different economic system, based on an environmental, humane, libertarian vision that exploits and shares resources.

Polyamory finds its place "elsewhere" in the logic of love, much as libertarian environmentalism finds itself "elsewhere" in the logic of politics and the economy. It is no coincidence that the former is gaining in popularity at a time when the latter is also making headway, at least on an analytical level. There are several striking conclusions that the two analyses have in common:

Nonappropriation: Environmentalists refuse to accept gene patenting and appropriation of living species. Polyamorists refuse to claim ownership over the people they love.

Respect for natural cycles: Environmentalists advocate the respect of animal reproductive seasons and cycles. Polyamorists call for the respect of the cycles of desire, which are far from being linear. For them, the idea of breaking off a relationship simply because it is going through a dry period is as ridiculous as the idea of chopping down a tree in the winter simply because it has lost its leaves, forgetting that after winter comes spring. Of course, they are no more exempt from the pain of romantic breakups than the next person, but they make such decisions after mature reflection and not as a result of pressure from ruling hormonal, passionate impulses.

Biodiversity: Environmentalists believe that monolithic solutions—be they in the auto, nuclear, or genetics field—are doomed to fail and lead only along the path to dependence. They feel rather that it is far more sensible to approach the future by opening up more possibilities. Likewise, polyamorists believe that monogamy sterilizes love and fosters unhealthy codependence, whereas multiple relationships feed off of each other's differences and ultimately lead to enriching fulfillment. Polyamory aims to find a balance between stability, wherein children are not made to bear the brunt of their parents' emotional ups and downs, and a need to grow emotionally, intellectually, and sexually with lovers who bring their individuality to the table to the benefit of all.

The importance of bonding: Environmentalists warn that a society based on performance and competition can only harm social bonding and have detrimental effects on our attentiveness to others. Along these same lines, polyamorists do not focus on sexual performance and transcend the boundaries of romantic rivalry. They nurture emotional relationships where words, caresses, attention to, and interest in the other take the place of expectations and performance requirements.

This meeting of principals between environmentalism and this "ecology of love" called polyamory leads us to the same conclusion. It is widely accepted that to create a livable society for all and a sustainable environment for the earth, small gestures are not enough; the need to change our global outlook on the structure of the world is becoming more and more urgent. Similarly, in order for it to find its identity, polyamory cannot merely move over to accommodate a monogamy which would, at best, condone romantic relationships outside of the couple. What is needed is a new take on love, freedom, and the responsibility that every person has over his or her own life. A clear, yet flexible system. However, like any major shift, there must be many stages. One becomes polyamorous over time, through asking questions and affecting micro-changes that eventually lead to a completely different way of life, just as some environmentalists, by first sifting through the debris that surrounded them, have managed to find a space where they can live happily and comfortably far away from the sirens of overconsumption.

QUESTIONS

1. What is the hardest part of abandoning the model of monogamy?

It is exactly that—abandoning the model—that is the hard part! Even though this way of life may seem restrictive, it is always comfortable to live within the norm and fairly easy to step outside of it with discretion. To stand up and live openly outside of that norm, on the other hand, exposes you to the reactions of others, which can at times be quite aggressive. Added to that is the fact that every day involves a journey down an unknown path, where rules and reference points need to be reinvented as you go. Many men, initially drawn to polyamory, will renounce it not as the result of moral conflict, but for the simple fact that adultery is easier. On the other hand, women, if monogamy has not been too entrenched in them, are generally attracted to the idea of polyamory, which they greatly prefer over adultery. They admire its openness, clarity, and the fact that genuine relationships take precedent over mere sexual encounters. Since the publication of *Aimer plusieurs homes* (*To Love Several Men*) in 2002, the concept of polyamory has come a long way, particularly among young people, who see it as a refreshing alternative to the divorce culture of their parents' generation. It is discussed in books, in internet forums, and on websites,[10] bursting the bubble of isolation in which many poly men and women feel they are

---

10 Such as *www.polyamorysociety.org* and *www.worldpolyamoryassociation.org*, among others.

confined. This now being the case, their lives should get a whole lot easier in the future.

2. Why try polyamory when it's so easy to cheat on my partner discreetly?

Polyamory is not an excuse for adultery! It is a life view based on the responsibility and autonomy of the individual. For poly men and women, romantic diversity—in fact, diversity in general—is preferable to singularity as it allows an individual to express many parts of his or her personality and heightens self-confidence, intellectual curiosity, and creativity. Sexuality is but one of many areas through which these traits are fostered. The decision to become poly often comes hand-in-hand with the launching of other projects that are important to both men and women, like changing careers, learning a new craft, or traveling. Their new take on love and relationships, by kicking out the old system of thought that had repressed them for so long, liberates them from prior fears and gives them the energy to take the leap into a new life.

3. What is the difference between polyamory and the sexual liberation of the 1970s?

Polyamory incorporates sexual liberation, but its logic is different and its philosophy more global. The sexual liberation movement of the 1970s, under the banner of "free love," was a reaction to the prudishness of previous decades and entered the scene as a literal explosion of the senses. However, given the climate of intense politicization, sexuality did not escape the clutches of ideology. The expectation of sexual liberation was almost as widely enforced as that of monogamy. Its roots were not desire but an ideological need to reject "bourgeois" jealousy and embrace the breaking of the taboos and shackles of yesteryear. Moreover, it was merely tacked on to previous patterns of behavior without allowing individuals the time to really analyze their sexuality. Quickly, then, we saw the emergence of macho instincts, of men imposing their desires on women with complete disregard for their own. This, in turn, provoked a feminist response whereby everything that represented this masculinity was met with hostility.

Polyamory operates under a much more egalitarian ideology, where individuals profit from freedom without being forced to express it: A poly man may go through periods where he has no partner, where he has several, or where he is monogamous, but he remains a poly man, free in his romantic conduct. Poly women are feminists who love men: comfortable enough to have no need to exclude or defend themselves against this half of the population, sure enough of themselves to not be afraid to love.

4. Is polyamory the same as swinging?

Polyamory certainly allows for partner-swapping but sets itself apart from the standardized model of swinging, in which seduction and sexuality reign over the importance that polyamory gives to the creation of relationships. Besides, liberation through swinging remains theoretical in nature, as swingers are open only to an exchange of partners within sets of couples, and a male partner may refuse to share his partner with a single man (or the other way around). Furthermore, many swingers forbid emotional ties between sexual partners, as well as personal encounters outside of the couple, which runs contrary to the philosophy of polyamory.

5. Can poly men and women be single?

Absolutely. Polyamory is a personal choice before it is the choice of the couple. In theory, single poly men and women have no limits to their personal freedom as they have no one to answer to and no expectations to fulfill. In practice, however, things are not so simple. Single poly men and women may find themselves up against demands of exclusivity or the constraints of jealousy and may, sooner or later, ask themselves if the time has not come to share their freedom and build a life with a long-term partner. Single poly men and women impose the same limits of respect that anyone owes to his or her partners. The questions that come up in this book do concern couples for the most part, as it is in applying a romantic practice that runs contrary to this structure of ownership of a partner and sexual exclusivity that problems occur. However, let it be clear that the suggestion here is not to enforce polyamory in place of monogamy, but rather to expose people to the wide range of possibilities available so that they may chose their path, both in love and in life in general, with an open mind.

6. Why is it that couples that get divorced, remarry, get divorced again (successive monogamy), and so forth, are considered faithful, whereas polyamorous couples,

who have long-term and even life partners, are considered unfaithful?

Private life must mirror society in order to be accepted. A few generations ago, when one entered the service of an employer and remained there for one's entire life, the monogamous couple corresponded directly to this idea: one job/one boss, one marriage/one partner. Economic crises and an increase in divorce rates exposed the fragility of bonds that were previously believed to be everlasting, as well as the dangers that appear when one puts one's survival—be it economical or emotional—in the hands of a single structure. The habits of attachment, however, are hard to break. People prefer to sever ties, make new ones, then sever them again and start from the beginning. Our current period could be defined as a time of sentimental and professional channel-hopping, whose consequence is the anxiety of instability and whose collateral damages lead to repetitive disruptions: material losses, displaced children, repeatedly broken families, and so on.

7. Is polyamory, like sex-toys or communal living were at other times, just a trend?

"Polyamory" and "multiple relationships" are words that are heard more and more, and we may therefore have reason to believe that the subject could become a media trend. Some people will give polyamory a try . . . and fail . . . for it requires such a rethinking of one's preconceptions in relation to love, that one must first be sure that it is the right thing to do in order to persevere.

8. Why does polyamory provoke such adverse reactions?

Polyamory offends people because it answers their questions in a manner that is logical and coherent, yet at the same time completely contradictory to dominant strains of thought. It accepts the realities of desire without hiding behind the myth of "one love." Its model is open-ended and forms itself on the free will and independence of the individual. Its approach is revolutionary and secular: "Live as you see fit, without imposing your beliefs on others," which runs contrary to the overbearing fundamentalist trend currently sweeping through societies today.[11]

Polyamory sees sexuality as a privilege, a joyful means of communication, unlike the guilt-provoking prudishness and constraints of standardized sexuality. It advocates peaceful and responsible romantic relationships in societies where dramatic breakups and crimes of passion have become commonplace. In addition, it creates perfect equality between men and women.

Freedom, equality, secularism, respect: when all is said and done, polyamory is an ideal life choice for a democratic republic. Furthermore, in many countries, more and more couples are now opting for civil unions in place of marriage, which constitutes a contract between loved ones who wish to build a life together, without necessarily demanding sexual exclusivity.

---

11 Take, for example, the increased influence that churches enjoy in the United States, and the rise of fundamentalist Christian groups in the EU. "Thema," *Arte*, December 2008.

Love

Love! A feeling surrounded by questions and anxieties when it could be so simple: be seduced by somebody, delight in their very existence, revel in their happiness, cry at their grief, and be there for them in their time of need. Love would be the most liberated, altruistic feeling there is—if we didn't insist on chaining it to the shackles of obligation ("If you love me, you must do this . . ."), unrealistic demands ("Prove that you love me!"), and anxiety ("Is this feeling really love?").

I lose count of the number of women who write to me about men with whom they enjoy making love, talking, and sharing countless things, yet ask themselves, for the simple fact they are not eaten away at by anxiety, "Do I really love him? Does he love me? Is this really what they call love?" Wrapped up in the fantasy of the tragic romance of literature, with all of its flamboyance and excess, they let wonderful men simply slip through their fingers. This downfall is certainly more feminine in nature than it is masculine. A woman's need for love is more powerful than her desire for a man. One such woman spent the evening telling me about a man she had been dating, a man so handsome he had women falling at his feet. She was overjoyed that he asked for her phone number over everybody else, but complained that he was obviously not keen enough, given that he had waited two days before calling her. I couldn't help but ask her if she loved him. "Yes, I think so. I think about him a lot, anyway." "I'm just asking," I told her, "because for all the talk about how much you want him to love you, you haven't told me one single thing about him, about what his interests are, or what he does."

What is the most common criticism that people have about poly men and women? That they don't know how to really love. Why? Because they enjoy independence, they are not eaten up with anxiety, they reflect before breaking up a relationship, they know how to spend the night with a lover without necessarily making love, they accept that their partner can love somebody else, they can cancel an intimate date if their child is ill without having to worry that their lover will take offense, and they are capable of being apart from a lover for months while still feeling for them deeply. As a result, numerous attempts to affix the correct label to their feelings have been made: is it love, desire, indifference, frustrated passion, or seduction?

One of the most difficult steps in reprogramming the "romantic central nervous system" is to be sure to not label feelings by giving one priority over another. Mothers do this naturally: while they love their children in different ways according to their individual personalities, they do not love one more or less than they love another, except perhaps in very rare cases. Poly men and women shy away from this form of labeling, as life has taught them that relationships evolve in cycles, with high and low points, and that to endeavor to box them into any particular category would be in vain. Sometimes we love our partner as a friend, sometimes we cannot stand her, and at other times we are overcome with passion for her. The same goes for all men. The question is, why should we bother putting a label on relationahips when life seems intent on peeling them off, without losing sight of love?

QUESTIONS

1. Why does love start off so well, only to deteriorate over time?

Romantic relationships begin in a narcissistic fashion: What gives the ego a bigger boost than knowing you can please and seduce somebody? During this phase, one is concerned more with oneself and the effect one is having on the other, rather than with the other as a person. It is also a virgin phase, like the first blank page of a notebook for scribbling dreams and fantasies. The dream of love is often more enticing than the person himself/herself during this phase. Next comes the editing process, when dreams meet reality. Just as a manuscript with a few words scribbled out is proof of a work in progress and not of failure, so the scribbles in the "man-uscript of love" show an evolving bond and the discovery of intimacy. The passion experienced at the beginning is not conducive to the ensuing needs of work, raising children, forming friendships, and cultivating interests outside of the relationship. Therefore, it is a good thing that this initial phase eventually winds down. Nature dictates that the initial hormonal rush responsible for passion slowly dies down after two or three years. Unfor-tunately, the extent to which we are seduced by novels and fairy tales in which love is synonymous with passion leads us to lament the fact that things are not "like the early days" without acknowledging that, had it remained stuck in this preliminary phase, love would be fixed in a state of paralysis.

2. Why do men find it so difficult to commit to love?

Most men will one day want to find someone with whom they can share their life and build a future, one that often involves children. However, this desire goes hand-in-hand with the fear of losing his freedom and being shut out at the doors of the possibilities life offers. Day to day language does not do much to reassure them, with expressions such as "getting hitched," "being tied down," "taking on the old ball and chain," and the like. This fear of being so limited often puts them off the idea of living as a couple, unless they can find a partner who will accept their desire to live polyamorously. They find themselves accused of a fear of commitment, something they would happily embrace if it did not go come as part and parcel of the confines of romantic exclusivity.

3. Friendship + Desire = Love?

When things are going well in a friendship, you do not question how long the relationship will last, whereas this is a recurring anxiety when passion comes into play. But if desire comes along and attaches itself to friendship, what more could you possibly ask for? More importantly, why feel the need to label the feeling?

4. How do I know which love is true love?

Only at the end of our lives will we know whom we really loved and who really loved us. It is quite possible that we will have had more than one defining relationship. Nevertheless, certain bonds are unique: that which is shared with the father or mother of one's children, for example, as the latter will depend on their parents for their entire lives, and those parents, polyamorists believe, sign up for a lifetime of responsibility. Therefore, selecting a mother or father for one's children is more important and more delicate than choosing a lover. Another unique bond is that which is built up over time: to know someone for ten, fifteen, twenty years, or even more creates an attachment that is wider than just romantic feelings, and is only made stronger by years of shared experience, much like a tree trunk is strengthened each year by an extra ring of bark.

5. When we talk of "couples" and "polyamorous relationships," is there not an assumption that the latter ranks lower than the former on the established hierarchy?

Many poly men and women begin with a vision of a main planet—the couple—surrounded by satellites.

Over a period of years they discover that polyamory is an individual choice rather than the choice of the couple, as it is not necessary for both members of the couple to be polyamorous, so long as the choices of the poly partner are accepted by the other. Polyamory considers each relationship to be unique, void of hierarchy and rivalry. Some bonds, however, do take precedent over others, as discussed above, and relationships dominated by an all-consuming passion do not fare so well over time.

6. One lover told me that he didn't want to fall in love with me because he didn't want to get hurt. Am I destined to live a life of "good friends," without the spices of passion?

This might be the case, if it were not for the fact that passion comes knocking when you least expect it, and poly men and women are just as susceptible to its charms as anybody else. On the other hand, though, they are less likely to make decisions under its influence, preferring to wait for it to run its natural course before making any important choices. That said, some men find it hard to open up completely with poly women, or feel unable to fully accept their romantic freedom. They punish them, as it were, by convincing themselves that it is the sexual and not the emotional aspect of polyamory that attracts them. Others say that they fear being hurt and so maintain a certain distance in the relationship. This reluctance fades over time, and many men who were not initially keen on the principal come to relish the joy that poly love brings.

7. Friendship, complicity, intimacy, partnership, desire . . . is it possible to find all of these things in one man?

It is perfectly possible to find these things in one man . . . and also in many others. With a life partner you can find yourself lovers one moment, family the next, and friends the one after that, depending on the circumstances. During a fight you may feel that he is your enemy, and you may simply experience indifference in moments of weariness. But this is what keeps the fire burning, for if everything was predictable, you would quickly lose interest. In this way, a lover with whom the only connection is sexual will soon become tiresome, whereas a friend could arouse desire when you least expect it. To put someone into a category—like acquaintance, friend, or lover—is to disregard the other sides of that person's personality. By breaking down these boundaries, polyamory dispels preconceptions and allows for the possibility that someone you thought you knew so well could suddenly surprise you.

8. Does polyamory apply to homosexual couples?

Polyamory operates outside the confines of sexual orientation. Homosexual men are often not exclusive, even with a partner they refer to as their "husband." Much like those who embrace polyamory, these men enjoy friendships through which they can share sexual pleasure and also activities and common interests. Playful sexuality is often an important part of homosexual culture, if the tell-all confessions of some are anything to go by. Partner equality, a concept fundamental to polyamory, is also important to many homosexuals, who claim that their sexuality is much fairer than heterosexuality. Partners may take turns assuming the role of penetrator or penetrated, dominant or submissive, which runs contrary to most heterosexual relationships, in which few men enjoy the roles of penetrated and/or submissive. However, jealousy and power struggles exist in homosexual relationships, which often fail to escape the clutches of dominant morality, even though the mere fact of their sexual orientation offers them an easier way out. The ostracism and marginalization that has been forced upon them for so long, and continues to be to a certain extent, often leads them to firmly assert their identity outside of the social order that rejected them. The vision of some homosexuals falls more into the category of swinging than of polyamory when it comes to sexual relationships.

Preconceptions

"You can only love one person at a time. . . . Jealousy is the proof of love. . . . Men have more sexual needs than women. . . . He's the man of my life. . . . A single love is so much more beautiful. . . ."

Hypothetical love is packed full of statements of this type, statements we accept without question and on which we base our emotional lives despite the daily contradictions offered by reality. The 10 percent of men who actually admit to leading a double life—there are surely more, but many prefer to keep the secret—know perfectly well that they love both partners.[12] Any monogamous man who will one day have a lover knows that he is capable of loving his wife and his lover. "It's not the same

---

12 This figure according to a survey published in the French publication *Francoscopie* (Gérard Mermet).

thing!" you will hear him cry, and he is right. That every love is different, that chemistry between two given people is unique, is precisely the reason for which polyamory is so enriching. One relationship does not rate higher or lower than another, but rather they are different, complementary, and for this reason, non-competitive.

Which brings up the issue of jealousy. Is jealousy really the proof of love? Consider the fact that the majority of domestic violence cases and so-called crimes of passion are caused by jealousy. Is killing somebody one claims to love, rather than seeing that person happy elsewhere, really that beautiful a way to express one's love? To treat the other person like an object of possession! Isn't true love about wishing the other person happiness, wherever it may be found?

"Men have more sexual needs than women. . . ." Letters I have received and audience secrets revealed during programs on sexuality show that the female libido is just as alive and kicking as its male counterpart. Furthermore, how would men satisfy these vital needs if there were not so many women ready to respond to their desire? Men themselves understand and dread the romantic ardor of women: a little-known book by Dr Gérard Leleu, *La Mâle Peur* (*Male Fear*), shows that men have been trying to restrain the female libido since ancient times, be it through circumcision, the veil, or strictures of "feminine decency," as they put it. As a result, women have been driven to disguise their desires, but not for one moment has the flame gone out.

"The man of my life" is one of the more persistent preconceptions, thanks to fairy-tale promises of a Prince

Charming who will whisk his princess away and protect her from all evil. Some women are so convinced that this man exists—a man who will bring 100 percent satisfaction to them and them alone—that they spend their whole lives looking for him. From divorces to separations, they do not realize that they may have passed by two, three, four, or perhaps more "men of their lives," a clear demonstration that "the one" was merely an illusion.

As for the notion that a single love is more beautiful, it simply does not hold up in the face of reality. The vast majority of monogamous men and women have been in love more than once in their lives, either before or after their marriage, and cannot even answer the question, "Why is loving one person better than loving several people?" As one poly man put it, "The concept of one love is evil, because it forbids you to love anybody else."

In the void between the reality and the myth of love is born a sentiment of frustration and failure, and myths certainly have a tough time of it. To accept that love is not as we are told in films, novels, and songs is painful, just as it is painful for a child when he or she discovers that Santa Claus does not exist.

Polyamory is anything but myth. Basing itself on the facts mentioned above, it envisages a romantic life that is not an illusion but a fulfilling reality. Rather than suffer the void between dream and reality, polyamory embraces reality and builds its own dreams. [13]

---

13 This was illustrated by an Anglican pastor in a report on infidelity on the French television channel Arte: "Man has given himself the impossible objective of loving only one person in his life, and suffers on a daily basis from the fact that he cannot meet this goal."

QUESTIONS

1. Why should I never be able to so much as look at another man just because I met my husband when I was twenty years old?

The simplicity of this question highlights the absurdity of some people's preconceptions. If you lived to the age of eighty, or perhaps more, how could it be possible that not one single other man would be worthy of your desire or your love? You met a man (and probably a handsome one at that!) at the age of twenty, but he represents a minute percentage of the number of men who will cross your path during your lifetime. Would it not have to be quite a mighty miracle if he were really "the one"?

2. I fell in love with a colleague and we are now lovers. People have always told me that "looking elsewhere" is a sign that a relationship is failing, but I love my partner and have no desire to leave him.

Why should loving another mean that you no longer love your partner, when you seem so perfectly happy? There is a chance that your relationship will end at some point, if the day comes that you no longer have anything to share. But if it does, then this end will come whether you are monogamous or not. It will have nothing to do with meeting other men, but rather with the fact that you will have reached the end of your road together. The notion that you must leave one relationship in order to begin another hurts not only the partner who is left behind, but also the partner who moves on. And that is without even considering the possibility of children being involved.

3. My male friends dream of having multiple relationships but claim that their partners wouldn't be able to handle it. My girlfriends dream of such relationships too, but say that their partners are too jealous to accept the idea. Who should I believe?

Everyone thinks they are right, and this is partly due to preconceived notions of men and women in general, and more specifically those of our partners. One reader, a fan of *To Love Several Men*, decided to try sharing the book with his partner, sure that she would throw it back in his face. To his great surprise, she confessed that for many years she had been thinking of such a lifestyle but had not known how to broach the subject with him. There is still a long way to go with communication between men and women. . . .

4. Ever since I revealed that I'm poly, it's all people will talk to me about! It's hard to be judged on this one aspect of my life, without credit or interest being paid to the other things that interest me.

The act of judging and cataloguing goes way back, particularly in France, where people who live outside of the norm are seen as freaks of nature. Take Régine Desforges, a novelist and cross-stitch artist, as an example. She also participated in countless political debates, but to this day she is thought of as a publisher of scandal and an erotic writer. If this label bothers you, then be discreet about your polyamory until the time comes when it is commonplace enough to no longer incite unhealthy curiosity.

5. My therapist doesn't agree with polyamory. He says that it's a sign of emotional immaturity and that it is impossible to love more than one person in anything other than a superficial way.

Therapists are no more exempt from social conditioning than anyone else, even if they have spent time studying it. Some may offer exceptional help to their patients while at the same time suffering devastating divorces or pathological family conflicts. The therapist to whom you refer is confusing love with passion. A lot of people would find it very mature of you to want to preserve a stable family environment for your children without renouncing your romantic life, whereas people who go through successive monogamous relationships drag their innocent children through spirals of conflict, divorce, and broken families. It is not the place of a therapist to judge your behavior. His or her role is to help you untangle the way your mind operates in order to be aware of your strengths and weaknesses, and to consider them when making decisions in the future. If a therapist is making you feel bad about yourself instead of better, the best thing to do is to find another one.[14]

---

14 I would like to take this opportunity to thank Dr. D. Thanks to his objective and benevolent ear, over several months I was able to accept myself for the person that I am.

Independence

Benoîte Groult offers two definitions of romantic independence in the following statements: "Share what can be shared, but let each person live his life as he/she sees fit," and "Love is when two people remain just that until the end of time." This notion may run contrary to the myth of the inseparable couple, but it is certainly in keeping with reality. Even those of us who are surrounded by friends and are loved by many are born alone and will die alone. We also suffer alone, for no matter how well our loved ones take care of us, physical and mental suffering cannot be shared. At the funeral of a parent, brothers and sisters are comforted by the warmth of their family bond, yet each grieves in his or her own way. Grief is as unique as every parent/child relationship and, further, any loving bond.

An independent person is able to deal with life situations on his or her own: acceptance and rejection, joy and sadness, doubts and certainties. It is also vital to honor the independence of others by accepting their choices, by granting them responsibility for their own happiness, and by not feeling guilty in the eventuality that you do not live up to their expectations. As children, we aim to please our parents in order to win their love, driven by the fear that if we are not the sons or daughters of their dreams, this love will be revoked. As adolescents, we break away from our parents in an effort to create our own values, to burn the bridges of childhood dependence, and at the same time, albeit subconsciously, to test the limits of their love: "Will they still love me if I'm insolent, obnoxious, and worry them out of their minds?" Becoming an adult should be defined as being independent, staying true to ourselves, and being capable of loving others for who they are, never sacrificing our principals to please them, and never attempting to change them to make ourselves happy. It should also require that we be able to accept moments of solitude without a feeling of abandonment, and to reach out to others because we like them, not out of a fear of being alone. This independence is a must for a successful polyamorous lifestyle. It requires the marriage of self-confidence—"This is how I am. Period."—and respect for the other—"You are different from me. Period." When these two planets collide, we see the birth of love founded on understanding and not codependence. To reach this level of independence does require a certain amount of intellectual effort, so engrained in our way of thinking is the notion that love requires mutual dependence, a shared "wavelength," and that solitude is not only bad, but a social defect. The success of social networking sites, where users acquire "friends" (some of whom they have never met) at an alarming frequency, is a clear demonstration of this need to feel surrounded by loved ones. Best not to mention that even a user with 357 loyal "friends" on the screen is most likely sitting in front of that computer screen alone! Poly men and women are not antisocial—far from it—but they believe that while it is possible to benefit from the vital support of other people, it is on oneself that one must count in order to make it in life.

QUESTIONS

1. How can I avoid becoming too attached to a loved one?

Independence is favored over dependence in all areas of life. Professionally, if you work for a single client, you rely on them entirely for your financial well-being. If you work for several, then to lose one is not disastrous. Similarly, if you put all your money in one bank and that bank fails, you are ruined, but if you spread your investments around wisely, you will still have some of your savings left if one bank goes under. The idea is the same with love. If your love life is built around one person, then the void left by separation or death will be devastating. If you love more than one person, however, while a broken heart will still be hard to bear, you will know that you have other avenues of sentimental existence to explore. And it's not just a question of loss; if you live a poly lifestyle, you will see that dependence decides to make itself scarce, to the great benefit of your lovers. You are not with them because you need them, but rather because you love them, and you will not suffocate them with your desire for attachment.

2. Even though she doesn't say so, I feel that my partner resents me when I go out for the evening. She tells me I'm being ridiculous and to stop talking about it, but I can't help feeling guilty.

Perhaps you think she resents you because you feel guilty and believe that her happiness is your responsibility. Maybe she is not as interested in polyamory as you, but even though you wish it were different, that's her choice and you must respect it as she respects yours. If she says she doesn't want to talk about it, respect her decision. It is often the case that poly men and women get so caught up in their lifestyle that all they want to do is talk about it. Instead, try asking her about herself, her work, her plans . . . accept your differences and don't force her to enter your territory. Go toward hers for a change and share the things that excite her—perhaps they will excite you too!

3. How can I explain to my married lover that I feel guilty when she lies to her husband in order to see me?

There is certainly a guilty party in this affair, though apparently it is not you but she who is lying, and that's her business. Perhaps, knowing her relationship as well as she does, she feels that a white lie is better than the truth, which may devastate her husband. By understanding that every adult is responsible for his or her own choices, we are able to react to situations in a rational manner. A women who seeks revenge on the "evil temptress who stole her husband" often forgets that that husband was probably not forced. A lover who decides not to tell her husband must have her reasons, and you shouldn't judge her. Nonetheless, you should be able to talk about your discomfort with the situation with her.

4. My partner accepts my polyamory but has no desire himself to have other relationships. Can we live with this imbalance?

Bravo to your partner for the emotional maturity displayed in wanting you to be happy, even if it is not in a way that corresponds to his own emotional needs. This accepted imbalance is much more preferable than if your partner felt he had to force himself to have lovers too. Maybe one day he will want to do so, but until then, explore your romances with discretion and without guilt. When you go out, you don't have to say whether it is with a lover, a girlfriend, or work colleagues. Be considerate of your partner, and be sure to handle your passion and potential heartbreak without dragging him into it as well.

5. My partner enjoys our poly adventures but can't stand the thought of me forming a personal attachment to someone else. That, though, is precisely what interests me: having male friends with whom sex is a possibility, but not an obligation.

Many men feel more comfortable with swinging as a couple, as it allows them to spice up their sex life while still feeling in control of their partner. Your partner is afraid that he will lose his hold on you if you have a personal life. He is not embracing the spirit of polyamory, which is based on equal partner autonomy. Like many women, you prefer the ideals that come hand in hand with this way of life. It all boils down to negotiations between the two of you, the goal being to express your desires and your vision for a shared emotional future. The ideal solution is that each partner makes an equal sacrifice in order to find a compromise that suits you both. There are hundreds of ways to love more than one person, including the generic agreement: "Do what you want to do, but don't tell me about it." If the disagreement continues, then the choice is yours: leave the relationship in order to live in keeping with your deepest feelings, or continue in an unsatisfying relationship in order to avoid the pain of separation.

6. My lover said to me, "You're not independent, you're selfish." This statement really hurt me a lot.

Obviously this man, as Oscar Wilde before him, believes that "a selfish person is one who doesn't think of me." He is upset because he is not the only person on your mind. Are you selfish because you think of yourself? Because you live a life that suits you, even if it doesn't fit other people's image of you? Because you are full of *joie de vivre* and are in love with the idea of pleasure? Don't blame him, but ask him to explain his thoughts. Christ himself tells us to love our neighbors as we love ourselves—proof that to love oneself is essential, not selfish.

7. I spent two weeks alone this summer because my part-ner was on vacation with his lover, and my lovers, who are married, were away with their families. What is the point of being poly if I still find myself alone?

Polyamory doesn't guarantee that you are constantly surrounded by devoted lovers! In fact, the greatest les-son it teaches is that you can be alone without anxiety, safe in the knowledge that it is a temporary state with-in a constantly rotating cycle of love. Being alone can be quite pleasant if you get along well with yourself. Temporary solitude is mostly unpleasant because of the preconception we have of it, or that we imagine others having: "I am left here looking abandoned" is a simple ego issue.

8. Is it essential for a couple to be drawn to polyamory for the same reasons?

It is vital that both partners agree on the concept; however, one may be drawn to it because he enjoys the art of seduction, while the other is attracted by a curi-osity to discover different types of men. If one restricts himself to two lovers but the other spreads her wings a little further, it really doesn't matter. The important thing is that their polyamory satisfies them both without affecting the core of their relationship.

9. My partner has fallen in love with his lover, and this is unsettling our relationship. He seems distant, dreamy, even melancholic. Should I intervene?

It is not your place to make decisions for him, even if you're afraid that he will leave you. To intervene would stir things up unnecessarily. Let him follow the flow of passion for the moment, and concentrate on the things that interest you outside of your relationship with him. That doesn't mean that you can't remind him of his role in your everyday life; being in love doesn't give him the right to leave everything else to you, or to be away so much that you can no longer make the most of your independence, something that is particularly important if you have children. If he becomes hostile or indifferent, maybe it would be best to separate for a while. To enjoy his newfound passion is one thing, but to make you pay for it is quite another. You can be understanding of your partner's behavior without having to accept every part of it. You have the right—in fact, you owe it to yourself—to fix the limits of your own tolerance.

Coming Out

To tell or not to tell—the million-dollar question! There are valid points on both sides of the coming-out argument. On the "for" side, the very definition of polyamory—that desire for multiple relationships is expressed openly—means that it should be talked about. To live this love in secret would be the same as living with adultery. However, some readers of *To Love Several Men* have written to me with this ironic observation: "You are doing what everyone does. The only difference is that you're talking about it!"

Those "against" coming out believe that polyamory is a private agreement that does not concern anyone else, that things that are this intimate should not even have to be shared with loved ones, let alone in public. The other side reminds us that the gay movement had to stand up and make itself heard in the media, often in provocative ways, in order to begin to be accepted by society. In this way, if polyamory as a subject were to become more commonplace, it would no longer be shunned and blacklisted to such an extent.

The "against" camp, however, counters that society has an uncanny knack of exploiting new phenomena such as this. Take, for example, the trend of sex toys, which appeared on shelves at a time when women were demanding that their need for sexual pleasure be recognized. This was a perfect example of genuine reflections on feminine sexuality being turned into a gadget commodity—to the benefit of sales, of course. These critics also predict that it would not be long before poly clubs, cruises, and parties would emerge onto the scene . . . bringing with them themes of swinging and classification forbidden from the beginning.

On the "for" side again, it is worth considering that poly men and women often feel isolated and misunderstood, and would take comfort from the knowledge that others think and live as they do.

The debate is far from over, and opinions depend greatly on the varied environments in which those concerned live. It is easier, for example, to confess to being poly in a staunchly liberal family than within a community of fundamental Catholics. At the end of the day, no one is obliged to tell all about their life. However, the more men and women speak out about polyamory, without preaching, the more it will be taken for what it is: a way of loving people that is not harmful or immoral, but joyful and responsible. For this to happen, honesty is an essential tool, but one must have enough self-confidence to stand up to problems caused by the unhealthy curiosity and snide remarks that may ensue.

Thanks to friendships I have formed since the publication of *To Love Several Men*, I tend to lean more toward the "for" camp, whereas criticisms and exclusions that I sometimes suffer as a result of coming out have a habit of pushing me back toward the side of those against. It is clear that this question is something that must be decided on a case-by-case basis.

QUESTIONS

1. How should I approach my parents, brothers, and sisters about polyamory?

The family is an emotional refuge but also, sometimes, a place of violence. Families are made up of tightly woven intergenerational threads, which include old conflicts, rivalries, and the unique bonds formed by blood ties. And then, of course, there is the even more complex issue of step-families. It can be futile to bring a potentially explosive subject to the table of a family already filled with resentments. Your love life is your business, and you do not need the consent of your family, nor do you need to rub your rebellion in the face of their convictions. Older generations or religious relatives could be overcome with shock at a sexuality without taboos, given that they themselves have suffered at the hands of such limitations. On the other hand, if you have a peaceful, trusting relationship with your family, then you may want to share your experiences on this subject, just as you would with close friends, without having to explain every detail of your intimate life.

2. My partner wants me to explain to any lovers I may have that we're poly, because she can't stand the idea of being seen as a pitiable victim of infidelity.

Her request is perfectly understandable, if only because you should be being honest with your lovers. At the same time, you don't have to subject them to a lecture on the ins and outs of polyamory! Just explain that you and your partner have multiple relationships without lying to each other, while still exercising a certain level of discretion. No lover is going to like the idea of you giving your partner a detailed run-down of your exploits every time you get home!

3. It doesn't seem very elegant or enticing to explain to a man immediately that I'm poly. When should I tell him so that he doesn't feel like just another number on the list?

In all likelihood he'll ask you fairly early on if you have someone else, if you're married, if you have children . . . any man and woman will want to get to know each other when they first meet. You could put it this way: you are faithful but not exclusive; you don't believe in a Prince Charming, but rather that there are many men out there worthy of getting to know better. That should be enough. If the questions persist, if he demands that you tell him how many lovers you have and wants details, run away! This is not the behavior of a gentleman. If one of your lovers falls head-over-heels for you and wants to marry you immediately, it would be better to be open and honest from as early a point as possible.

4. How should I talk to my lovers about the other men in my life, be they partners or lovers?

You don't have to talk about them. As long as they know about your lifestyle, the rest is not their business. Would they like it if you told other men about them?

5. My partner knows that I have other lovers. My lover, on the other hand, refuses to talk to his partner about it, and he feels extremely guilty. Shouldn't he be honest with her?

Things are always easier when every player is open and mature about their outside relationships, but this is rarely the case, as polyamory remains the choice of the minority. It is for your lover alone to decide whether he would prefer to live with the secret and guilt, or to come out and run the risk of hurting his partner. As for you, don't try to persuade him one way or the other—it's not your job to lead his life. If the guilt he is dealing with becomes difficult for you and affects your relationship, it would be better to take a little distance, at least for a while.

6. I have been invited to take part in a television show about infidelity. I'm torn between the desire to go and get things out in the open, to help move them along a bit, and the fear of how my friends and family will react.

If you are strong and are not easily affected by the way that others see you, if your family is open-minded and your workplace non-conformist, then why not give it a go? If not, it might be better to decline the invitation, as television has such a huge impact that it can have far more serious repercussions than we initially imagine. Also—and I speak from experience—the very fact that the word "infidelity" is being used signifies that the program is based on the dominant train of moral thought, which makes sense, seeing as television is mostly geared toward the majority. But that means that by going on the show, you risk being marginalized, attacked, caricatured, and given only a few minutes to explain yourself and a complex lifestyle. In staged debates, it is very difficult to be heard, and everyone has a role to play; I have come out of some shows looking very wrong-headed, while others happily rattled off moving stories about fidelity and the joys of an exclusive love that has lasted for more than twenty years. (For the record, many of them came along to my dressing room afterward to thank me for my words and to confess the truth of their real love life! The audience, of course, was unaware of this.) Given the fact that most shows are pre-recorded, the editing process can leave you saying things that are the opposite of what you intended to express. Televised coming out is a very dangerous exercise.

7. Neither our families or friends know that we are a poly couple, but I enjoy keeping a blog of my romantic endeavors (changing names and places, of course). This was not enough, however, to prevent one of my lovers from recognizing herself. She is furious and is threatening to kill me!

The internet is like a breeding ground for words, and they can turn around at any moment and attack their creator. Anonymity can also not be guaranteed. You don't have to be a computer expert to trace a source and identify the blogger. The golden rule of the internet is discretion—especially if you have chosen to live a life that is hidden from your friends and family! Avoid blogging about your encounters—it is unfair to your lovers, even if you present them in a flattering light. Jealousy aside, they may wonder whether you are interested in them for who they are, or because you want to look like a stud in your blog. If the urge to write is too much to ignore, then try writing fiction, where you can mix facts, people, and places with elements of pure invention—without running the risk that people will recognize themselves. As for the lover who is threatening you, stop seeing her and change your phone number. And don't forget that it is dangerous to let a woman believe she is the only one, if that is not the case.

Trust

Trust is essential for a polyamorous lifestyle. I have been contacted by many a reader in a state of panicked urgency: "My wife has gone off with a lover and left me with our three children! I am devastated!" or "I've just found out that my husband is in love . . . with another man! I'm crushed and don't want to lose him." After meeting these people, it was clear to me that their shock stemmed more from the fear of being abandoned and lied to than from the affair itself. Women in particular have a keen eye for deception. A change in a partner's behavior may indicate that he has a lover, and the woman is almost relieved when, after bombarding him with questions, he finally confesses. This relief comes because they have left behind fantasy and suspicion and entered the stage of reality.

Things are always more difficult in our imagination than they are when we actually deal with them. This wisdom can be seen in the cruelest of all losses: death. When we think of the eventual death of a loved one, the imagined pain seems so unbearable that it would not be possible to survive it, and we are unable to even allow ourselves to believe that it is a possibility. However, when the unfortunate event arrives, as it does in all human life, we go through the usual phases of grief: denial, anger, sadness, and eventually peace. Much like the time that the first stage of romantic passion takes to run its initial course, grief takes around three years to overcome.[15]

Similar phases, although shorter in length, are experienced with adultery. The partner who discovers it feels as though his world has been turned upside down and is unable to believe that such a nightmare could possibly be happening. Then, presented with the evidence, he becomes angry. Some stay stuck at this stage, which is a major reason for so-called crimes of passion. The one who continues on the road of reflection will experience a feeling of deep sadness that comes less from the love that his partner feels for someone else than from the fact that he has been lied to, that feelings have been hidden. He feels humiliated and is shaken by the fact that he built his relationship on foundations that are now crumbling: "I trusted her completely, and she betrayed me."

When asked, "Can you accept that she was able to feel desire for somebody else?" eight times out of ten

---

15 Consider the lyrics of Jacques Brel: "On n'oublie rien de rien . . . on s'habitue, c'est tout" (We never forget a thing, we just get used to it).

the response is positive, accompanied sometimes by a cheeky smile: "I understand because I too have been chatted up and have had to force myself to not give in to the temptation . . ."

The root cause of this pain is a double question of trust. The trust that the cheated person put in the other, and the trust that he put in himself, a self-confidence wounded by an event that has proven that he is not in absolute control of his life, even if other things—work, plans, health—are doing just fine.

Polyamory requires that one works on and develops these two types of trust, which must first of all be better defined. Mutual trust, as some define it, does not necessarily require complete transparency and disclosure. These demands are more a sign of a lack of trust, given that they imply absolute control over what the other person does, says, and thinks. You can only learn to trust someone in stages: at first it is essential that there be a dialogue surrounding what each person is feeling and how things are to be structured. It is a must that any feelings of apprehension and concern regarding the new romance be expressed to the other partner. At the same time, it is important that there is an understanding from the beginning that each partner respects the other's privacy and accepts that some things be left untold.

Learning to trust and have confidence in oneself is equally complex, as the education and social systems condition individuals to recognize their faults rather than their abilities. Starting as early as report cards: "Could do better . . . "; "A good semester . . . try not to let it slip in the next one . . ." These loaded phrases, which lead us to believe that we will never be quite good enough, never commended unconditionally, never loved for our complete selves, weaknesses and all, set the stage for a chronic, lifelong lack of self-confidence. According to many psychotherapists, the majority of depression cases and behavioral problems can be blamed on a lack of self-esteem. It creates resentment, introversion, jealousy, and even arrogance as a tool in a desperate attempt to be noticed by others by being overly assertive. Is it possible to love others if we do not love ourselves? Christ himself responded in the negative. The cultivation of a gentle, humble sense of self is an important part of the poly learning process. Fortunately, this process is not learned in textbooks but rather by following the path of experiences as they occur.

As I describe in *To Love Several Men*, the first time I saw my partner with a lover was accidental, and the mere fact that I came out the other end of it unscathed was the first building block of my self-confidence. I have been cultivating it ever since, breaking down apprehensions that risk inhibiting my life choices one by one. As I wrote then, "Before that night, I would never have thought that such a thing was possible, but there I was—alive and not a hair out of place. Quite the opposite, in fact: I felt a enormous sense of self-confidence of the kind one often feels after surviving a difficult ordeal." The further into polyamory one gets, the more self-esteem one builds in the discovery that what once seemed insurmountable, even unbearable, was, in the end, not that big of a deal. Sexual non-exclusivity is not deadly, after all, and is actually quite trivial compared to some of life's other difficulties, and global events that shake the world in which we live. On the contrary, the feeling of self-confidence gained from one's own poly relationships, and the mutual trust that prevents one from feeling let down or disregarded as a result of one's partner's relationships, are key to feeling genuinely happy.

Polyamory, by accepting the reality of plural desire—a reality recognized by most monogamous people, even if they do not act upon it—and by refusing to live these desires under the camouflage of humiliating lies, allows both partners to trust. These desires are not uniquely sexual, or uniquely emotional or intellectual. Poly men and women embrace this sentimental complexity, which brings them closer to those they love. In so doing, they nourish their partners' feelings of trust by refusing to pacify them with naïve illusions and degrading lies, like "It was just one night, honey. . . ." This learning process is not something that can be achieved in a single day, but the required effort is well worth it. Such a level of trust and confidence makes all aspects of life easier and greatly reduces stress and anxiety in the future.

QUESTIONS

1. How can I build up my self-confidence so that I no longer doubt myself (I'm not good enough, or not beautiful enough) each time my partner has a new romance?

Every new relationship brings with it doubt and mystery, which is completely understandable. This would no longer be a problem if you stopped comparing yourself to other women. Instead of thinking of yourself as more or less beautiful, intelligent, or sensual, you must accept that these women do have some things you don't, just as you have qualities that they don't. You are not rivals but are merely different and complementary to each other. Coming to this understanding takes time, but you will get there. Tender, satisfying moments that you share with your lovers will help to boost your self-esteem. By seeing that this feeling is possible, you will no longer feel anxious each time your partner spends time with someone else.

2. My partner wants me to tell him every detail of my relationships as a sign of the trust we have in each other, but I believe I have a right to my "secret garden."

Demanding to be told every detail is not a sign of trust but of control. Trust exists when two people agree to accept that each keeps an air of mystery, which in addition can fuel desire. If this desire is lacking these days, despite a profusion of studies on sexuality, it is perhaps because in over-talking the issue of sex, we have removed this indescribable element that feeds it. Besides, a detailed rundown of erotic exploits can be unhealthy: exhibitionist on the one hand, voyeuristic on the other, or just plain annoying—even if he's not jealous as such, it's not always pleasant to hear your partner talk about how wonderfully she makes love to other men. Contrary to other manifestations of sexual liberation, polyamory respects the secret side of every person and the right to pleasure without informing the rest of the world or allowing them to watch from the sidelines.

3. How can I explain to my partner that she can trust me, that I am capable of desire for another woman without risking our relationship?

You just explained it perfectly. Of course, it's much easier to do it here than face-to-face with your partner, when you would have to defend yourself against challenges like, "If you love someone else, you must love me less," or "You want to jump on anything with a skirt, is that it?" Sitting opposite a woman who dreams of being "the one" for you and is insecure at the slightest idea of competition, the conversation is not easy. You may discuss the same thing a thousand times without her hearing what you say, because her understanding is inhibited by a fear of abandonment and/or a possessive instinct. Assuring her that your lover will not put your relationship in danger will only beg the retort, "How do you know?" And, truth be told, you don't know, because you've never tried. The only way of finding out whether multiple relationships can be natural for you and your partner, and can coexist without drama, is by giving them a try. Try responding to that effect: "Well, really, the only way to be sure would be to try." That may work if she has a sense of humor . . .

You could also give her a copy of this book, or, if you have friends who are openly poly, invite them over and discuss it together. In a relaxed atmosphere, your partner may warm up to the discussion.

4. How can I trust my lovers when the whole idea of the relationship is that there are no rules or obligations? I'm afraid of being taken advantage of.

They are taking advantage of you, and enjoying you, just as you take advantage of the ease and simplicity of your relationships. Do they still want to see you even though nothing obliges them to do so? That should be enough to allow you to trust them . . . and yourself.

5. My lover's wife sets rules that he can't wait to break with me. How can I believe that he isn't breaking the rules that I set with someone else?

You can believe it, but you can't be sure. Love is a game of uncertainty and uncontrollable impulses. Give him the independence to set his own rules if we're talking about games. If you believe he's breaking an important one—for example, that he's not using protection with his other lovers—then confront him about it to avoid anxiety in the future, or make him take HIV tests at such a frequency that he will find it easier to protect himself.

6. I trusted my partner completely, but discovered years later, despite our agreement to be poly, that he lied to me on several occasions. Since then I find it difficult to make love to him.

You are one of many women for whom trust is a sexual release. To have lost this trust has stopped you from letting yourself go. Your mind may whisper that the lies were not as serious as all that, and your heart may have forgiven your partner for his sins, but your subconscious is blocking your body. If you are still happy together, then it doesn't really matter: sexual harmony may resurface over time, or take second place to your emotional and intellectual bond. You could try re-sparking things with some sexual games or erotic conversations that, little by little, will help build a new intimacy between the two of you. Your poly lovers could also help to fill the void. However, if sexual relations with your partner are important to you, then only by working through your problems, perhaps with the help of a therapist, can you break through the blockade.

7. I feel like a dog who can't attract anyone. How can I possibly imagine multiple relationships when I don't seem to be able to attract even one person? Polyamory is a luxury for the rich and beautiful.

It can't be denied that rich, beautiful, and healthy people are generally favored over the poor, unattractive, and unhealthy, and not only when it comes to love lives! This inequality has no place in polyamory; in fact, it is quite the opposite, as love is considered as a pleasure that should be free and accessible to all. Further, it is often easier to please more than one person because, by putting fewer stakes on a relationship, you are more relaxed, carefree, and as a result, more attractive. Poly men and women's self-confidence allows them to be at ease and open, whereas people who do not love themselves have a hard time approaching others. There must be people around you who are not as beautiful or rich as all that with whom you can find fulfillment. It may even be the case that you will seduce a poly partner who is both rich and beautiful and who doesn't see you as a "dog"—don't forget that beauty is subjective.

8. At the moment, polyamory works perfectly for us. But what about fifteen years from now? Will I find myself alone while my partner continues to go out with younger women? I'm afraid of getting old.

Getting old scares everybody, but there is no choice, unless you want to die young. However, time is often kind to poly men and women, as a good dose of *joie de vivre* is better than any plastic surgery. In addition to this, they are less concerned with age issues, probably because their romantic relationships are not simply built on seduction, but also on profound affinities that are above the question of age. Also, contrary to the old misconception that men age better than women, the opposite has been the case over the last few years. Women in their fifties and sixties are full of life and charm, while their male peers are confronted with lower levels of desire and energy. The fidelity of poly men and women toward their past and present lovers provides them with a wealth of loved ones on whom they can depend, and with whom the stigma of time is erased by memories of golden years gone by. Despite the wrinkles and the slightly less-firm muscles, through an infrared gaze that transgresses the years, old feelings can be rekindled, rich in the memories of the first meeting and enhanced by those that have come since.

Guilt

Judeo-Christian society has been living under the veil of guilt ever since Adam and Eve were banished from their earthly paradise and condemned, one to hard labor and the other to painful childbirth.[16] Eve was punished for succumbing to the Serpent when he tempted her with the Fruit of Knowledge. The Serpent is a rather obvious phallic symbol, and the story of Adam and Eve a representation of the desire to keep the woman in a state of ignorance and to make her afraid of her sexual curiosity. In many polytheistic traditions, sex is joyful and even sensual, be it Hinduism with its *lingam*

---

16 It is interesting to note that in the Bible, work is depicted as a punishment (the French "*travail*" is derived from the Latin "*tripalium*," an instrument of torture). And the earthly paradise is a place where people are naked and happy!

(phallus) and *yoni* (female sexual organs) omnipresent in the erotic statues of its temples, or Greek mythology and the escapades of Zeus, Bacchus, Artemis, and many other sexually adventurous deities.

There is none of that in monotheistic religions: Just before they are banished from the Garden of Eden, Adam and Eve look at each other, become aware of their nakedness, and feel shame, to paraphrase the biblical text. And so we see on what pedestal the monotheistic West places its collective unconscious: the guilty woman, shameful nudity, and forbidden knowledge that is reserved for God alone—God being masculine, of course. As for the Serpent, he is at once fascinating and frightening, just as the phallus is for many women.

Whether you practice a religion or not, it is next to impossible to not be influenced by culture and history, and with a heritage such as this it is no surprise that polyamory, based on principles running completely contrary to religious dogma, poses a threat equal to that of the Serpent itself. The woman finds herself free, pleasure is enjoyed without shame, and both sexes can discover each other in an open, fulfilling context. As for the phallus, poly women embrace it not with fear and reverence, but rather with love and sensuality. And all of this without an ounce of guilt, for polyamory does not hide itself away, but stands up for its values in peace and openness. Poly women are not the sort of women who collect notches on the bedpost, nor do they castrate lovers or steal husbands. They enjoy natural, open relations with men, and it is precisely for this that they are blamed. If they lowered their eyes and begged forgiveness when admitting these liaisons, if they blamed lust and passion for their deviances and expressed shame, or, even better, if they were overcome with grief and regret, then society would happily forgive their behavior and put it all down to the weak constitution of the female sex. Poly women, however, are perfectly healthy in both the moral and physical sense, and see nothing wrong with using their bodies and intelligence to express love to men, who are themselves also beings endowed with body and brain. Period.

As for poly men, considering society's abhorrence of male infidelity and the misery inflicted on their wives—so extreme that laws protecting women, particularly in matters of divorce, are based on the hypothesis that sooner or later a man will abandon his wife and leave her penniless as he starts a new life with a younger woman—to admit to a lack of guilt is more than a little tricky. And then of course there's the notion that adultery is nothing but a sexual impulse, confirmed by so many men who claim that they and their mistresses are no more than mere ships passing in the night. But polyamorous men—they speak of love! An unforgivable sacrilege. No mercy is shown to these poly men who "destroy the homes of others" and poly women who "clutch at men with their witches' claws, dragging them off to fulfill their perverted fantasies."[17] To deny that these lovers are capable of acting under their own free will is to completely discredit them. It is possible in any romantic relationship,

17 I hope that readers will forgive this rather vulgar and pompous language: these are word-for-word quotes used in letters that I have received.

no matter how passionate, to distance oneself or break away if things start to turn sour. Poly men are the first to admit the dilemmas that their lovers may face, but they refuse to make decisions for them and consider them to be entirely responsible for their own choices.

"I am responsible but not guilty." This famous statement by Georgina Dufoix during the contaminated blood scandal was mocked by many, but the point she made is not really as ridiculous as all that. Guilt as a sort of self-punishment is an unmistakably Judeo-Christian trait and is not necessarily synonymous with responsibility. For example, it is quite possible to feel guilty for defrauding the taxman without actually accepting responsibility for it. On the flip side of that coin, the director of a vacation resort could be held responsible for an accident that happened to a child, even if he was not at fault in any way and the child hurt herself as a result of her own carelessness.

This subtle distinction is highlighted in the case of a relationship in which one partner leaves the other after an affair about which he/she feels guilty. It would be more responsible to accept the desire that led to the affair, which may only be short-lived anyway, without breaking up the home; to see if it stemmed from a lack of something within the relationship, or from an exquisite lust for life; to let things run their course and see where they are heading. In order to do this, one must accept that desire is not something to feel guilty about, but rather the essence of life, something positive for one's own existence and not a negative for that of the other person. Or, if someone is not at a point where this paradigm shift is possible and still feels that his/her behavior is wrong, then those feelings of bad conscience must at least be accepted and not taken out on the other person, like the men who blame everything on their "she-devil" wives in order to absolve themselves of their own guilt.

Because poly men take responsibility for their own decisions and suffer no guilt as a consequence, they are quite capable of explaining to another man the reasons for which they love his partner. From here we find situations arising that would seem surreal to a monogamous couple, such as an evening meal where a man finds himself at that table with both his partner and a lover, with all three discussing their feelings openly. Or perhaps a meeting between a couple and the wife's lover, the purpose of which is to iron out problems that are causing an imbalance between the different parties. A further example would be a woman calling her lover's wife to ask for advice regarding the love she feels for the latter's husband.

I have even been sent "family" photos, where partners and lovers pose around the same table. In order to reach such a point of harmony, it is essential to come to terms with the fact that pleasure is not a guilty feeling, but nor does it give you the right of ownership over another.

It is hard to believe that a war built on the lies of one country,[18] the pillaging of poor countries, the job losses of millions of workers, the failure of the financial system, or cases of tax evasion produce less of a scandal than the

_____

18 The famous Iraqi "weapons of mass destruction," to use one example.

statement, "We each have simultaneous, multiple relationships, and we're happy about it."

QUESTIONS

1. My partner and I are on the same page in terms of our poly lifestyle, but I still feel guilty when I come home after a wild night . . .

Your reaction is understandable. The Judeo-Christian philosophy that is so entrenched in our minds considers pleasure a sin and glorifies the notion of sacrifice. The fact that you choose to put yourself first—especially if your partner then spends the evening alone—is bound to bring up feelings of guilt, but these will die down over time as a balance is reached through which you can both be happy, whether together or apart. At that point, things will feel so natural that you will wonder how they ever seemed so complicated. The feeling of guilt is not as altruistic as it seems: feeling guilty is a sign that one feels responsible for the happiness of others, as if they were unable to manage that themselves. Omnipotence is the sequel to desire.

2. I feel that I should be more affectionate than usual toward my wife after a night out. Does this mean that I feel guilty?

Possibly, but it could also be that you are grateful for the opportunity to live freely and happily, and you want to express that to her. Make sure that she appreciates your affection. Even if she didn't believe it at the beginning, she'll soon find out that polyamory does great things to her husband!

3. I only date single women because I can't stand the thought that if I am with a married woman I may be hurting her husband. The problem is that being married myself, I feel guilty when I return home to my wife and leave my lover alone.

Whether the married man is openly poly or acting behind his wife's back, things can always get complicated with secret lovers who sit by the phone, waiting for it to ring. But they will certainly suffer less with a man who is open about his intentions to love them but at the same time doesn't lie about one day marrying them, and doesn't lead them on in the belief that he is preparing to divorce his wife. Be loyal and honest with your lovers, and let them get on with their own lives.

4. After discovering that we had both been unfaithful, my husband and I have decided to be openly polyamorous. I feel less guilty, but I've lost that thrill that came from having illicit affairs.

You belong to a group of women who take pleasure from transgression and guilt, and who yearn for forbidden sex. To spice things up, try inventing erotic games with your husband or lovers where you play the role of a guilty woman, with some kind of punishment as a bonus. Try making love in places where you risk being caught by strangers, or coming up with other forbidden scenarios that will fulfill your desire to disobey. You must also remember that just because you've decided to embrace polyamory, you don't have to tell your husband about every encounter, nor the extent of the feelings that may ensue. In that way you will be able to keep a little of your mysterious side. . . . Does that idea excite you?

5. Intellectually I agree with polyamory, but the idea of my boyfriends practicing it makes me anxious. In my family, when a man cheats on his wife, he leaves her. How can I move beyond the beliefs that my education and religion have instilled in me?

It's hard to conquer those beliefs completely, but they can be tamed over time, much like overcoming a phobia. To attack a negative condition head-on is an exercise in futility. You will wear yourself out trying to discuss the ins and outs of polyamory with a man who believes that a woman is his property. Opt instead for more simple relationships, through which you can enjoy meeting other people without hurting anybody. You will discover, bit by bit, that you're not alone in this way of thinking. With poly men you will experience warm, problem-free relationships and will overcome your fear of polyamory little by little. The men in your family may have left the wives they cheated on in order to escape the complications and scandal brought on by adultery. If they had been able to stay with their family and love other women at the same time, they probably would not have left. The majority of men are deeply attached to the idea of family and the notion of the couple. Moreover, many poly men re-enact the couple model within their parallel, outside relationships, whereas women tend to look for a way to escape this convention—where they are often saddled with the majority of material chores—through polyamory, which presents them with playful romantic adventures and offers a balance to their daily lives.

Desire

Polyamory is a manifestation of desire in the psycho-analytical sense of the word. The power of this desire can be compared to the concept of Qi in martial arts: a life force so strong that it banishes inhibitions and allows for dreams to be realized. The discrepancy between life as it is lived and as it is dreamed is one of the major causes of depression. Interestingly, the first sign of depression is a loss of desire: the libido and desire to make love disappear, followed by the desire to do other things, and, in extreme cases, the desire to live.

To find a way to keep hold of that desire and live one's dreams—the founding principals of polyamory—would therefore be an excellent way to combat depression. But first of all, those true desires must be identified, a task much easier said than done, given how difficult it can be to separate one's real self from that imagined and hoped for by others. Young people are often thrown into the professional world without being fully aware of the track they are on or how they got onto it. A good student attends Advanced Placement classes, a lower-achiever stays back a grade. The first heads off to an Ivy League school, the other to mechanics classes at the community college. The first marries a young female engineer; the other, the girl next door. The first becomes CEO of a multinational corporation and hires the second to work in his factory. At the age of forty they both discover, perhaps after a period of depression or a heart attack that causes them to reassess things, that they never really chose their path in life.

This digression may seem far from our subject of romantic freedom, but it is interesting to note that poly men and women often decide to live this lifestyle after an existential crisis forces them to reevaluate their lives and to ask themselves whether they are really what they had hoped they would be. The freedom to love that is embodied by polyamory—not to be understood here as merely unbridled sexuality—leads us to question other ways in which we have been conditioned over the years without really realizing it. If you have always been led to believe that jealousy was an uncontrollable, primal feeling, but it turns out that you can control and live with it after all, then what does that mean for the other feelings you have been suppressing? That said, the ups and downs, doubts and complications encountered by poly men and women keep them in touch with the reality that the path to fulfilling one's desires is not an easy one, nor does it necessitate the complete destruction of all former reference points. Contrary to some monogamous individuals who abandon their families from one day to the next because they have found love somewhere else, poly men and women assess the role of dreams and reality in their feelings, and respect their commitments and priorities. They exist in the midst of joyful romantic spontaneity and cautious clear-sightedness, which leads them to think before they act, something generally uncommon, and not only in matters of love.

It goes without saying that not all poly men and women reflect on things to this extent, and that some people embrace this life style solely because they enjoy multiple relationships without complications. What I describe here is the product of thirty-five years of reflection. There are many intermediate stages and many different ways of life, but each one merits our attention if its aim is to stimulate, and not condemn, the energy of desire.

QUESTIONS

1. Is it not dangerous to follow the whims and rhythms of desire when desire itself is so uncontrollable?

What you're talking about is the passionate sexual desire of a new relationship. It is indeed dangerous to make important life decisions under its influence. For this reason, when I find myself faced with a lover who is crazy about me (and I think the word "crazy" says a lot here . . .), my standard response is that, while I am ready to enjoy the whirlwind aspect of the relationship, I am unwilling to make any life commitments until at least two years have gone by. Some people leave immediately upon hearing this, but it has been my experience that the majority stick around and become long-term lovers.

2. If nothing is forbidden, how can I stimulate desire?

Poly men and women don't necessarily think of "the forbidden" as being a stimulant. What excites them is curiosity and a desire to discover the various ways in which individual lovers express themselves and to uncover different aspects of their own personalities in relation to those lovers. Their desire comes from their ability to experience passion as a magical moment, something otherworldly, which takes place "on the other side of the mirror."

3. How can I tell if the desire I feel toward somebody is genuine, or if there is a hidden agenda that even I am unaware of?

Every desire has hidden agendas to some extent. Even though polyamory defines desire as a genuine interest in and an irresistible attraction to another, this desire can still contain subconscious motives. It can reassure a person that they still have the charms to seduce. It can be a tool in the quest for a balance of power within a poly relationship, where one partner seeks to test the limits of tolerance proclaimed by the other. It can fill a sexual void or compliment one's daily life. It can arouse hidden aspects of an individual's sexuality that were previously buried in the subconscious. But the fact is that it doesn't really matter if desire is not as altruistic as polyamory would like to have it. The important thing is to be aware of this, and to analyze your thoughts in such a way as to not be blinded by your feelings, and so as not to mislead your lovers.

4. How can polyamory help me to embrace other forbidden desires?

Polyamory frees us from the preconception that we can only love one person at a time. It shows us that this preconception is built on fear, on possessive, controlling instincts, or on the need to satisfy our inner narcissist, but not on desire and even less on love. Once you make the breakthrough in understanding that the thing of which you were afraid, the thing that seemed so impossible before, is perfectly within your reach and can be a source of great pleasure, there is nothing to stop you from taking on your other inhibitions and discovering whether the things that were holding you back were doing so justifiably or not. Let this Buddhist phrase become your personal mantra: "Believe nothing until you have tried it yourself."

5. Isn't there a chance that you will get tired of having sex if you do it every time you feel like it?

We get tired of sex when we do it without desire. Polyamory is not about incessant sexual overconsumption, but about adapting one's sex life to one's true desires. Sometimes these desires are multiple, sometimes single, and sometimes nonexistent. A period of wild, frequent love-making may easily be followed by a period of abstinence or sexual exclusivity. And that's where real freedom lies: demands of sexual fidelity are not replaced by demands of promiscuity, but rather by freedom based on the respect for one's desire and the desires of those with whom it is shared.

6. I have a lover whom I see every Tuesday. Since I felt myself falling in love with him, my desire has only been decreasing! It's not like it was at the beginning, even though we haven't changed a thing.

This routine stems from the fact that you are dissatisfied with the relationship, something which is giving you the contradictory impressions that it is not as it was at the beginning, yet that nothing has changed! What draws you to each other aside from physical attraction? What do you do together? Any romantic bond, as wildly sensual as it may be, must also be nourished by shared moments and intellectual exchanges. It's not the sex that causes this routine to form, but rather your lack of common interests, and the fact that sex has been your only communication method since you met each other. If a relationship is to stay alive, it shouldn't be like the first day all the time. Maybe this man has nothing else to offer you, and so the relationship will fizzle out by itself; perhaps your meetings will become fewer and further between; or perhaps you will break up, only to get back to together at a later point. Poly men and women don't just walk out on each other; they recognize that a relationship is going through a tough patch and take the opportunity to pursue other romantic interests while life sorts out the rest.

7. How can I get through these periods of libido loss and fatigue, during which I just don't feel like making love to the men I care for?

Polyamory fosters bonds that far surpass sexuality. Keep seeing each other anyway and don't forget that you can still enjoy certain levels of physical contact and tender caresses if you feel like it. Warn your lovers in advance about your libido issue, that you're going through a bit of a "dry patch." As long as they don't feel rejected or responsible for it, they are likely to be open and accepting. If some of them don't want to see you platonically, then they'll take a little distance until your desire returns. Desire moves in cycles and must be allowed to recharge itself once in a while before making what can often be quite a surprising comeback. Keep in touch with your lovers during this time—words are essential in maintaining a bond and should be seen as a form of verbal caress, whose erotic power should not be doubted.

8. How can it be that my libido is heightened, even with my partner, since I have been seeing other men? Shouldn't I "get my fill" more quickly these days?

It's often said that eating only increases appetite! On a more serious note, your libido is obviously enhanced because polyamory has freed you from previous inhibitions and is allowing you to fulfill your fantasies. You've been reassured of your seductive powers and feel like more of a "woman" than ever before. As for "getting your fill" . . . desire and appetite are two different things. You won't die of starvation if you don't make love for a while, but nor will you suffer from indigestion if you do it all the time! Desire doesn't come knocking at the door at any particular time, and its different manifestations are controlled by the brain, not the sexual organs.

Variety

Variety is widely understood to be a quantitative notion. This would define polyamory as the compilation of a list of lovers and a pretext for sexual overindulgence, which is a mistaken notion. Polyamory is opposed to singularity in the same way that environmentalism is: "The world would not be where it is now, David, if it were not for the scientists, writers, builders, farmers, adventurers, dancers, and even the cops and the grocers with their gray overalls and their pencils behind their ears. For life to blossom, we need to live a variety of romantic experiences and should not hang our existence on one single being, brilliant as he or she may be."[19] Poly men and women may well consider that each love is unique,

---

19 Excerpt from Simpère's *Les Latitudes amoureuses* (*Latitudes of Love*).

but it does not follow that they believe that one love holds the answers to the entire universe, nor that they would claim to solely fulfill each of their own lovers. In other aspects of life this is quite clear—would anyone believe that they could satisfy their cultural appetite with just one book or piece of music? But when it comes to the subject of love, we find ourselves hung up on the issues of power and appropriation mentioned earlier. It is not so much the idea of having sexual relationships outside of the couple that is problematic for many—just ask the 40 percent of partners who commit adultery—but rather that these relationships are free and open.

Another aspect of the "variety" present in polyamory stems from the way poly men and women handle the ever-evolving components within their relationships, where the only rule is the mutual respect of each other's desires. A further source is their interest in each lover's way of life: a poly man or woman is like a sponge that soaks up unknown sensual pleasure. They love to travel, to learn, to discover new interests, and to embrace new projects, thanks to the lessons they take from their lovers.

"So you're talking about friends, then?" retort those who understand perfectly the richness of these bonds in friendship, but not in love. Yes, we're talking about friends . . . friends who share sexual pleasure if desire dictates, as a way of furthering the communication they enjoy. "Conclusion" is not an obsession of poly men and women. For them, sex is the beginning of a new kind of dialogue rather than the goal of a carefully orchestrated seduction.

QUESTIONS

1. If you multiply your number of lovers, don't you risk forming superficial relationships?

It is wrong to believe that poly men and women spend their time collecting conquests. Some have fewer romantic affairs than couples who claim to be monogamous! Polyamory accepts that during a lifetime, one will be attracted to many people, and that there is nothing wrong with acting on it if the attraction is mutual. If it seems that poly men and women have a lot of lovers, that is generally because they are loyal and maintain contact, at various frequencies, with the majority of the people they have loved. Some meet in high school and know each other as students, husbands, wives, divorcées perhaps, and then parents and grandparents. Their bond may sometimes be older than those they share with their official partners.

2. How many relationships is it possible to have at one time?

If you tend to lean toward sustained romantic relations, which demand that you spend a lot of time with each person, then you will naturally keep the number fairly low. If you have long-lasting relationships where frequent contact is not necessary, then you may have more, just as it's possible to have many friends without seeing them on a weekly basis. Some relationships will be put on hold as a result of moving homes, getting married, or any of life's other circumstances, and perhaps be picked up again at a later point. Others will be fleeting.

Given that polyamory is still the choice of the minority, some lovers may not stick around because they won't feel that they can handle the lifestyle. The question of "how many" is therefore not a pressing one; the response will come naturally in relation to each individual's life. One equation is more problematic: that of a man—more often than a woman—who feels split between his partner and his lover because the two relationships are not different and complimentary but rather similar and potentially competitive.

3. Are poly men and women really just selfish, focused solely on satisfying their own desires?

Of course some will be selfish, just as in any cross-section of the population, but in my experience, poly men and women tend to be attentive parents, natural lovers, and are curious about everything: art, politics, spirituality, travel . . . as if the fact that they are free from unnecessary romantic anxieties allows them to be open to everything else. Polyamory stimulates love for all aspects of life. If *joie de vivre* is selfish, then polyamorists are selfish, but given that feelings of happiness are contagious, it follows that they bring happiness to those around them much more than if they were grumpy and sullen. [20]

4. By spreading love around, do we risk it thinning out?

Desire, like love, is not a commodity that is taken away from one person if given to another. The desire

---

20 A scientific study in 2008 showed that a person's happiness and positive attitude are greatly beneficial to their immediate friends and family.

we feel toward one person won't be the same as what we feel toward another. The first will not be affected by the second, unless you only succumbed to the charms of the second because your desire for the first had run dry. The opposite can often be the case. Your libido, dulled after a period of inactivity, may undergo an awakening, to the great benefit of your partner as well as your lovers!

5. Are some people predisposed to polyamory?

The notion of predisposition implies genetic determination, and, it's true, scientists have tried looking for the unfaithful gene just as they have tried for that of the homosexual. The "infidelity gene," as it was hastily named by its Swedish researchers, is found more commonly in singles, men with mistresses, and, yes, polyamorists, than in those living exclusively monogamous lifestyles. But with a closer look, we see that this so-called "infidelity gene" actually has nothing to do with sexuality, but expresses rather an attraction to all that is novel, and a broad intellectual curiosity. It would probably be found with considerable frequency in researchers, artists, and designers. However, to admit to the existence of an infidelity gene, with all the derogatory connotations that come along with it, is not without harmful consequence. Imagine if scientists had summarized the study in this way: "Monogamous individuals can be characterized as lacking in intellectual curiosity and finding it difficult to adapt to change, whereas individuals who live polyamorously are genetically predisposed to express both of these qualities." The results would have had quite a different moral interpretation! Of course, environment also plays a vital role in romantic decisions: Young poly men and women today benefit from reliable contraception and sex information that was not available to previous generations, as well as the contributions of feminism and a desire to invent romantic ways of life that differ from those of their parents, who so often ended up in divorce.

If there is such a thing as a predisposition to polyamory, it is the consequence of these factors. The young independent son of divorced parents, full of curiosity and brimming with self-confidence, is a great candidate for a happy, polyamorous life!

6. Why look elsewhere when couples these days, thanks to the sexual revolution, are able to embrace all sorts of experiences, such as buying sex toys, for example?

Polyamory is not just about sex. Poly men and women don't "look elsewhere" because they are trying to fill a lack in their lives, but rather to meet others and explore their different worlds, sexual and otherwise. Desire is the fuel of our existence. This desire doesn't place much importance in sex toys, partner swapping, or gadgets, but dating, discovery, and curiosity are essential.

Equality

The notion of partner equality is by far the most innovative aspect of polyamory, and the hardest for many people to accept. Many Western democracies can show on paper that men and women have reached a point of equality, but reality proves that women are still treated worse than their male counterparts, both economically and within the structure of the family.

Polyamory is based on equality and refuses to accept that one sex dominates the other.[21] Women are granted the same rights, desires, and freedoms as men, but being equal, in this context, should not be understood as synonymous with being identical. Masculinity, femininity, hetero-, homo-, or bisexuality, and even androgyny are

---

21 With the exception of sex games, which do not cross over into real life.

important, but not defining, elements of each individual's personality, to be expressed as they see fit.

The fact that poly relationships do not operate within a hierarchy is another way they display their allegiance to equality. No relationship is better or more important than any other on a romantic level—they are simply relationships of a different nature, on different tracks. A relationship is formed around a shared life, which does require a certain level of commitment, but does not prevent each member of the couple—or couples, in the case of poly men or women who commit to future plans with more than one person—from remaining independent.

A perfect example of equality existing in harmony with everyday life can be seen in the case of a gay man I recently met. He was romantically involved with a man, but also with a woman who was soon to carry the baby he had always dreamed of. Alongside these relationships he was involved with his business partner, with whom he shared the running of their company as well as wild sexual encounters, and with several other short-term partners.

Is it utopian to believe that this level of freedom and equality can exist in love, a field traditionally rife with power struggles and dependencies? A priori, the answer is yes. But Utopia is a place worth visiting when you look at the extent to which it allows for stability and harmony within romantic relationships. And when the walls of this Utopia begin to overflow, as in the above case, it becomes a reality, one which does not aim to force itself on all, but to show that a different approach to love is possible, an approach that banishes violence and embraces joy and fulfillment.

QUESTIONS

1. Aren't men more independent than women—who are often jealous and sentimental—and therefore more suited to polyamory?

If the letters I've received and the reactions I've read in polyamory forums are anything to go by, it is actually the exact opposite. Women are drawn to polyamory because it allows for sentimentality within relationships, and because they are more than aware that men will experience multiple desires, a notion substantiated since the beginning of time by male adultery and polygamy in certain cultures. On the other hand, men, who may be enticed by the idea of a condoned adultery, are the ones that tend to find it difficult to leave behind their possessive instincts.

2. Why are some men uncomfortable, and sometimes even aggressive, if their partner is poly?

A lot of men fantasize about femmes fatales and seductresses but have a hard time accepting that the mother of their children could herself be this ardent lover of many. It's the old dichotomy of the mother and the whore. Men fantasize about their wife's desires and like to believe that they themselves can satisfy every last one of them, and can't help but wonder what another man could have that they don't. Virile male competitiveness continues to be a reality that is extremely difficult to uproot; it is hard for many men to accept absolute gender equality for which they must give up their ancestral domination. The young man of today, however, has come a long way on this matter. He recognizes that to be with an independent, self-confident partner is to be assured that she is not drawn to him out of material needs or psychological dependency, but rather because she considers him to be handsome, intelligent, and a good lover!

3. I am openly involved with several women and seem to have acquired a certain stud status! I know, however, that if I were a woman I would be criticized, even insulted for this. Is it not this gender equality that bothers people about polyamory?

Indeed, equality between men and women is a sensitive issue. Polygamy, practiced in many countries, is almost always a polygyny, which allows one man to have more than one wife, while polyandry, a woman having multiple husbands, is still quite an exception. Despite the fact that monogamy remains the legal regime in the West, many womanizing politicians and artists receive fairly good press, compared to a female singer with more than one lover who would be immediately labeled a "man-eater," in the derogatory sense of the word. Seductresses are easier to accept if they assume airs of scandal and show themselves to be outside of sexual norms.[22] But if, on the other hand, they go about the business of desire in a natural way, as many poly women do, without living a life of scandal, they are likely to intimidate some men, who are terrified of the idea that their partner could be seen in the same light as this other type of woman.

---

22 Consider the success of the book *La Vie sexuelle de Catherine M.* (*The Sexual Life of Catherine M.*)—Seuil.

4. My partner was unfaithful while I was pregnant. I found out accidentally and suffered a lot as a consequence. I managed to overcome my jealousy, and this made our relationship stronger than ever. Since then I find myself tempted by the idea of polyamory, but my partner doesn't even want to talk about it! I feel like I've been conned.

You have been, seeing as he allows himself the very pleasure he denies you. You demonstrated a great level of maturity in considering the reasons for his infidelity and turning it into something that strengthened your relationship. He has not done his part and is refusing to accept you as his equal. Polyamory can bring out fierce hostility in macho men who are dominated by the need for power. If your partner continues to refuse to discuss the issue, and especially if he becomes threatening, take a little distance to consider where the relationship is going, and don't be afraid to ask for help.

5. How should I handle things if I don't have a lover at a time when my partner has several (or the other way around)?

First of all, don't jump on the first man that comes your way in order to rebalance the equation, unless you find that man particularly irresistible! A poly couple is equal, but this doesn't necessarily mean that each partner should have the same romantic rhythms. If you are uncomfortable with this occasional imbalance, then talk to your partner about it—not to ask him to stay home, but rather to express how it makes you feel: lonely, insecure, or even jealous. He should take this into account when he plans his dates. If you prefer to make yourself suffer out of pride ("I won't let him see that I'm lonely") or on principal ("I don't want to sabotage his freedom"), then you must live with your choice. However, it's important not to force yourself to put a brave face on things, but to know how to express your weaknesses. We become stronger when we accept our limitations, and it is never a good idea to act thick-skinned if this is not the case.

6. Does respecting the principal of equality mean that I have to spend the same amount of time with each man?

Absolutely not. Equal is not the same as identical. Every relationship is unique, and there is no need for a standardized model. Live according to your desires, to your partners' desires, and to the free time you each have, while remembering that the feelings you have toward these men are the product not only of the time you spend together, but also the time you spend thinking about them in their absence.

Ego, Jealousy, Power

The countdown begins the minute we fall in love. We are happy, we feel safe, but the tender war has already begun. Couples who once loved each other so much that they yearned to live together and have children together are capable of pure hate when it comes to divorce, bringing out grievances that are sometimes more than fifteen years old. It's all well and good to speak of love and sharing, but the real con of the couple is the hidden fact that in joining together, each must lose a part of themselves, a part they will then stop at nothing to get back. But the costs are high, and the search can lead to daily confrontations with the other partner. Human beings have but one obsession: to know that they exist. The ego is a thousand times more powerful than love, and no one but the saints and Buddha are free from its clutches. And to succeed, the majority of them had to live lives of solitude.[23]

The inspiration for this emotionally charged monologue, taken from one of my erotic novels, did not just come to me in the middle of the night. It came, rather, from the story a friend of mine, who has since passed

---

23 Excerpt from Simpére's *Ce qui trouble Lola* (*The Trouble With Lola*).

away, and who dearly loved his wife throughout the forty-five years of their relationship. He told me that once, following a quite insignificant argument, that she unleashed a torrent of accusations against him, dredging up things that had hurt her as long as fifteen years ago. He was flabbergasted at the extent to which this women, whom he loved and who loved him, remembered grievances from so long ago with such frightening precision, as if she had known all along that they would be useful to her at some point and had deliberately stored them away. "We expect our enemies to be well armed when they finally declare war on us," he told me. "But your husband or your wife? It's terrifying! I was watching her as she spoke, asking myself: 'Does she love me or hate me?'" The answer was, most likely, both. The dynamic within some relationships can lead to confusion between love and hate, and family judges are paid to know to what extent a sometimes violent struggle for power can control the life of the couple.

This is not surprising if we look at the example of France, where the couple was defined by law as being fundamentally unequal. Napoleonic code granted single women certain self-governance rights, but considered a married woman to be under the full authority of her husband. It was not until 1946 that women were given the right to vote, 1965 that they were allowed to work and have a bank account without the written approval of their husbands, and 1967 that the Neuwirth Law finally legalized contraception. Clearly, female independence is still relatively new and is the result of decades of feminist activism and the fight for equality with men who ardently clung to their privileges. The female ego at that time? Denied. The male ego? Existing solely in relation to the domination of the other half of humanity, who submitted quietly, for the most part, in the name of love. The supreme entitlement of male/female relationships has, for centuries, been to lead women to believe that by losing themselves in love and giving in to passion, they are fulfilling a highly romantic, desirable destiny. Feminists, on the other hand, are depicted as "man haters," or, even worse, intellectuals.

It should be no surprise, in this context, that some women have become hostile toward men, and that some men, disturbed by the energetic demands of their partners, find themselves whimpering: "But what do they want?" and fueling the enterprise of magazines dedicated to masculine discontent and issues of manly identity.

Polyamory rocks this boat by favoring romantic bonds that are not based on male/female rivalry but on reciprocal desire between women and men in a setting of sexual equality, far away from the dynamics of ownership and domination. This is no longer a feminist revolution as such, nor is it one based on the idealization of love and the couple, but rather a battle fought by the combined, yet independent, armies of the female and male egos.

To win this battle, it is essential that both sides cultivate self-confidence and humility, signs of a balanced ego. The arrogance of megalomaniacs is generally a cover for a chronic lack of self-confidence. To be specific, self-confidence is when one is aware of his or her qualities without falling victim to false modesty, while humility allows one to recognize quietly that even though he or she is a wonderful person, there may be qualities that he or she lacks. An individual with a balanced ego is fully aware of his or her own existence and does not need others to confirm it. He or she is interested in others because of who they are, and not because of a need to see him or herself as a reflection in their admiring eyes. This is quite the opposite of what can occur during the stage of passion, where the important matter is the reflection of our idealized selves in the eyes of our lovers. Ego conflicts, often symbolized by jealousy, are the cause of the majority of problems experienced at the beginning of polyamory: it is sometimes hard to accept that one's partner has feelings that one is not a part of, to say goodbye to the omnipotence of which children and lovers dream.

Human beings are certainly not equal when it comes to the ego, which begins to form even before we are born: Neurological studies have shown that from the twenty-seventh week of pregnancy, the fetus' brain can pick up on the mother's stress levels and emotions, as well as the voice of the father. The emotional pedestal on which children are placed during the first few years of their lives, as well as their more or less stable, accepting social environment, play an important role in the development of self-confidence and a moderate ego. On the other hand, a lack or excess of stimulation, or an environment where any new experience appears potentially dangerous, can stunt the development of self-confidence and discourage intellectual curiosity and openness to others. However, we are all capable of overcoming obstacles, and as a result it is possible to control the ego and learn, little by little, not to allow it to control us. Polyamory is a great venue for this learning process, as it teaches us to understand that we are not unique, while at the same time reassuring us that we are important, through the creation of long-lasting, loving bonds. Further, it allows each partner the independence removed by the "couple," by returning to them the right to a personal life into which the other must not enter unless invited. Not only does polyamory embrace multiple romantic relationships, but also the ability to travel or go out alone, to pursue hobbies and interests independently, to not have to adjust to the other's biological rhythms (bedtime, meal time), and to not have to answer such questions as, "So, where have you been?" or "What are you thinking about?" In other words, the corresponding equation is $1 + 1 = 3$ (you + me + the relationship), and not the inseparable $1 + 1 = 1$.

QUESTIONS

1. How do ego problems manifest themselves in relationships between poly men and women who are in agreement on the principal?

Accepting the total independence of their partner is difficult for poly men, who have inherited a kind of ancestral machismo. Even if they refuse to express the anxiety caused by their partner's lovers, or if they try to trump their partner by showing that they're capable of having as many, or even more, lovers than she is, they often get locked in a power struggle, which is exhausting for all involved, and not in keeping with the spirit of polyamory.

For their part, poly women who lack self-confidence sometimes find it hard to believe that their partner is capable of continuing to love them as he falls for another, and constantly demand that he prove his love. They may sometimes throw themselves into the arms of another lover just to reassure themselves of their power of seduction, and to challenge their partner.

These difficulties will lessen over the years when time shows couples that if they've survived this many storms without a shipwreck, they should be confident in their life choices and sure of themselves. Not that conflicts won't still arise from time to time, but these couples will become more and more sure of their ability to overcome them, and will, more importantly, realize that problems are simply a natural part of any romantic relationship. They have learned to discuss, to distance themselves if necessary, and not to act on irrational impulses. They are able to listen to and understand the other's point of view, while knowing how to best express a contradictory opinion.

2. My partner says that it would disgust him to touch me, even days later, if he knew that I had been touched by another man.

Whether he knows it or not, his comment is a way of requesting: "Please, tell me nothing, never tell me if you have made love to another man," because he knows that his ego is not yet ready to accept it. This deep-rooted jealousy, which sounds as if it is hard to control, is based on the idea that female pleasure is in some way "dirty" and comes, perhaps, from the culture in which he was raised, or from his educational background. Some religions abound with references to impure women, whether they be dirtied by menstrual blood or by the attentions of a man. Perhaps these references have had an effect on your partner that even he is unaware of.

3. It irritates me to hear about my partner's exploits, and I have asked him not to talk to me about them. But he accuses me of being jealous, and even seems to get a kick out of it . . .

Your partner finds it difficult to understand that it is possible to love without being jealous, and your lack of jealousy makes him feel insecure. He is trying to provoke a reaction from you that may in turn reassure him of your love. You are perfectly within your rights not to want to hear the rundown of his romantic endeavors, which are part of his private life and not yours. Perhaps he tells you everything, under the pretext of transparency and trust, because he is angling for your approval in order not to feel guilty about his actions. Tell him that he doesn't have to tell you everything he does like a little boy begging for his mother's approval! Let him know that if he continues, you risk losing any desire you feel toward him, not because of jealousy, but because by forcing you into the role of mother and confidante, he is turning your love into an incestuous relationship.

4. When I watch my partner getting dressed up to go out for dinner with another man, I am torn between being

happy that she seems so radiant, and by feeling my heart strings tug just a little bit. Is this jealousy?

Of course it is, but it doesn't really matter. When your wife makes herself beautiful for an evening date, it's as if she is allowing you to read the first page of a wonderful book that she will then close, preventing you from reading the rest. It is normal to feel a little frustrated! However, your good poly nature allows you to be happy that she is spending a night of enjoyment and gratification. To delight in the happiness of our loved-ones, whether this happiness involves us or not, is to reach the core of polyamory, and it takes time to get there.

5. Why does my lover want to know if I'm seeing anybody else, when we always use protection and he himself has several other lovers?

His demand shows that ego issues don't only concern the couple, but also lovers. Your lover finds it much more natural to accept his own polyamory than yours! I'm sure that he would love to hear that he is your only lover outside of your relationship with your partner, or perhaps that he is your favorite. Maybe it would reassure him to know that when you are together, he is the love of your life, that the love you feel for him is unique even if it is not exclusive, and that placing your lovers in competition with each other is a romantic sport that you do not wish to partake in.

6. My partner decided to introduce one of his lovers to me. I was as friendly as could be, but she was quite the opposite. How should I have reacted?

You are in the dominating position of "partner," of "she who has been chosen for a shared life together." Until this point, you were an abstract entity to his lover, and she may even have fantasized about replacing you. When she saw with her own eyes that you were likeable and self-assured, she realized that she would never take your place, a place that she coverts simply because she doesn't have it! We always want what we don't have. There would have been no point in reacting to her poor behavior. However, the interesting point brought up by your question is that it is often wise not to mix family with outside lovers, as each inhabits their own world.

7. Why is it that my partner can't stand the intimacy that I share with a male friend, but has no problem with my lovers?

This question shows that the act of sex is not the only barrier separating forbidden relationships from permitted ones. The issue here concerns possessive instincts and the need to control. The love you feel for your friend seems strange to your partner because you are fulfilled without having sex. Platonic friendship between a man and a woman is unsettling for some men, because they can't help picturing themselves and the difficulty that they would have in resisting temptation, and actually fantasize about this mysterious intimacy. That being said, the ties that you form are your business, and you don't have to justify them. Everyone embraces polyamory in their own way. Other men would have more of a problem with their partner's lovers than with her male friends.

8. How can I tell if a man is really interested in me or if he just thinks that I must be good in bed?

You may not know at the beginning, but does it really matter? That first stage of seduction and desire is pure bliss, as long as you don't start fantasizing immediately about him being "the one." You'll know if he's really interested if the relationship continues, if you see each other sometimes without making love, or if he starts calling you just to see if you're doing well.

9. Is a poly woman a good or bad thing for the male ego?

That depends on the man and his self-confidence. Some men like a woman who plays hard to get, need this challenge in order to feel powerful, and are unsettled by a poly woman who doesn't fit that scenario and has no qualms about making the first move. A man who is only capable of imagining a monogamous couple, and is prone to jealousy, will also be caught off guard by a poly woman. Others, though, will be attracted by her *joie de vivre*, by her faithfulness to lovers as well as exes, and by the genuine interest she takes in each of the men she loves.

10. Thanks to my romantic experiences, I have really relaxed and made peace with the feelings that rattle my peers: unfaithfulness, jealousy, and breakups. I just can't take them seriously anymore!

Your experience has taught you to put things in perspective, which is a glorious thing. Unless the mild condescension I hear in your question is a subtle trap laid by your ego: "Oh, how much better I am than everybody else! I, the poly woman, who understands everything about love!" You must remember that everyone has their own romantic rhythm and works according to it in their own way. Their pain is real, no matter how petty it may seem to you.

11. When working on the ego, will there be moments of doubt and philosophical or existential questions that come up?

Not only will they come up, but it is extremely important to think long and hard about your agenda. Are you choosing polyamory because you are genuinely interested in the men and women you will be able to meet in an open and honest setting, or because you need to prove your sexual prowess by multiplying your conquests? Do you see polyamory as a lifestyle in itself, or as a way of feeding the illusion that you are living on the sidelines of society, that you're not like other people, that you are able to live a more intense life than anyone else? In other words, are you poly for yourself, or to outdo others? Are you genuinely happy loving more than one person, or does this lifestyle choice stem from a need to escape your daily routine, to make up for an emotional lack of some sort, or to pass the time? More bluntly put, are you in a state of genuine desire or Pascalian distraction? If you don't address these questions, you run the risk of future depression ("What was the point of it all?") or of living in the fear of growing old and losing your power to seduce.

Children

The issue of children is a crucial one for poly men and women. For a couple that has no children, wherein partners are in a position that would allow them to separate in the case of serious conflict, romantic freedom is deemed to be tolerable to a certain extent. Poly mothers and fathers, however, take this breaking-of-the-norms to a whole new level and find themselves asking, "How can we reconcile the respectability that comes along with parenthood and the images of debauchery and irresponsibility conjured up by romantic freedom in the mind of the collective subconscious?" The issue is also a crucial one for polyamorists because it forces them to make some pretty tough decisions. Imagine a woman who must decide which of her lovers she would like to be the father of her child, or a man who is not ready to be that father and therefore finds himself having to refuse his lover and deny her the child she dreams of. Gratifying lovers are not that hard to come by, but a man who seems to be good father material, even in the eventuality of future separation, is much more difficult to find. He needs to be a man with whom you can imagine sharing life's pleasures, of course, but also certain worries and concerns, for, as wonderful as children can be, they signify the end of carefree life as we know it. Our sole purpose becomes ensuring their happiness and protecting them from whatever life has in store for them, and the chosen father should agree that it is vital that adults do not allow the rollercoaster ride of their romantic desires to affect the lives of their children. In short, raising children is not something that poly men and women embark upon lightly: they are attentive, loving, non-possessive parents. They are not of the kind to vent their frustrations on their child, for the most part because they are inclined to not get frustrated in the first place! They allow their kids the independence that they themselves enjoy, while being there for them when the time comes. It is no coincidence that my mailbox has been known to overflow with photos of children and their poly parents, and that a large portion of the questions people ask me are on this subject.

QUESTIONS

1. Will men still find me attractive during my pregnancy?

Until your pregnancy is visible, they will find you as attractive as they always have—perhaps even more so, seeing as for the first four months your breasts will be considerably larger and you will have a certain glow about you. From then on out, some men may be less inclined toward sexual feelings, but others will be drawn to you more than ever, pregnancy being a sign of femininity and a powerful stimulant of desire. By the sixth month, though, most likely your own desire will begin to dwindle.

2. I recently gave birth and my attention is centered on the baby. Does having a child mean that my life of polyamory is over?

Perhaps for a time, yes, your romantic endeavors will take second place because you are wrapped up in the joys of motherhood. On top of that, you are tired from the birth, from a lack of sleep, and from being overwhelmed by everything that's going on. You will undoubtedly go through a period of mixed emotions, during which you will bounce back and forth between the joys of starting a family and the nostalgia for those wild years gone by, which suddenly seem a thing of the distant past. This dichotomy, which may lead you to believe that you've fallen into the trap you've been avoiding all these years, and that by making this one choice you have closed the door on many others, could cause you to feel extremely unsettled, something that those around you will not hesitate to label "postnatal depression." That is, until the day that you find yourself, to your great surprise, looking at a man with that certain wanting of days gone by, experiencing the impulses you thought would not return. Desire will come and go throughout your entire life. When you're more experienced with its whims, you will no longer be afraid of a loss of libido and won't think in terms of beginning, middle, and end, but rather of perpetual renewal.

3. Some of my lovers are already uncomfortable with the fact that I'm married. Will they have even greater uneasiness now that I am a mother?

Your lovers are uncomfortable with your husband because of the ways they identify with him. Particularly if they themselves are not poly, they tend to feel guilty that he is "suffering," given that he is experiencing something they know they would not be able to handle themselves. The fact that you are now a mother, though, will have quite the opposite effect by reassuring them that you're a real person after all, and you'll seem more approachable to them. It's a safe bet that your child won't affect your relationships, especially if your lovers are fathers themselves. You may even find that conversation will turn to your children and his, instead of their usual exclusive focus on your love life!

4. One of my lovers, who is worried about the ticking of her "biological clock," has asked me to father a child with her and swears that she won't ask me to be involved at all. I'm not so sure . . .

Your hesitations are justified—there is much more to having a child than getting a woman pregnant! Your lover's conviction that she will raise the child alone may be right for her, but what about you? How will you feel knowing that somewhere out there is a little boy or girl and you're the dad? Could you handle never seeing him or her? And if you get into a more long-term relationship, how would your partner feel about it? How will the child grow up, with only one parental figure, without ever knowing his or her father, which is quite different than having lost a father to death or separation? If your lover intends to find a partner at a later point who will help to raise the child, but has chosen you to conceive with either because she is in love with you or because you fit a certain desirable biological profile—health, medical history, beauty—the best thing to do is to run. A woman who has put this much thought and planning into her need for a child will get her way in the end, even if the man in question is quite clearly opposed to the idea at first. There have been enough examples of disputes of this nature to know that the best way to protect yourself is to cease having relations with this woman, unless she is already carrying somebody else's child. The only reason to accept would be if you feel strongly about having a child and that your partner doesn't feel the same way. You may well even decide to live and raise a family with your lover, while still continuing your relationship with your previous partner.

5. My partner is pregnant and doesn't really go out much in the evening anymore. Is it all right for me to continue my poly lifestyle?

Pregnancy is a very special, but delicate, stage in a woman's life. During this time she takes the biggest step of her entire existence: she moves from the state of being a woman, responsible entirely for herself, to the state of being a mother, responsible for both herself and her children, whom she will guide from infancy through adulthood. It's one of a few decisions that concretely involve the future: a baby becomes a child, an adolescent, an adult . . . and will always need his or her mother and father. It is understandable, then, that if a woman is conscious of this commitment, she may experience contradictory emotions during her pregnancy, swaying one minute toward jubilation, the next toward anxiety. During this time, poly women will perhaps put their lovers on the back burner for a little while, and this can be an added source of anxiety. In this case, you must allow your partner to decide on the rules: she may want you to spend more time with her, she may be happy for you to continue platonic relationships but not sexual ones, she may ask that you put your lovers on the back burner as well, just as the pregnancy has forced her to do. Respect her wishes for the moment; you can always come back to you romances later. It's quite likely that your lovers will empathize with your partner and encourage you to spend more time with her. The fact that polyamory favors the emotional and non-competitive aspects of love means that those involved, especially when it comes to long-term lovers, look out for each other, which leads to this kind, thoughtful behavior.

6. Should we talk to our children about polyamory? If so, how should we do it and at what age?

If polyamory is lived in a mature, open way, your children will be quite used to seeing their parents going out separately and talking about their boyfriends and girlfriends in friendly (and obviously not sexual!) terms. You don't need to give your children a lesson in polyamory in order for them to understand that their mom or dad is emotionally fulfilled. In the way that only children can, they will deduce that for themselves. As one of my daughters did when she was four years old: "So basically, you have Daddy and your boyfriends, and Daddy has you and his girlfriends." We had never specifically explained this to her!

7. My daughter would like me to tell her about my love life as she tells me about hers, but it makes me feel uncomfortable.

Even if you didn't feel uncomfortable, I wouldn't recommend that you tell her about your love life. There's no harm in telling her that you are involved with more than one person, and to even discuss issues of love, polyamory, and jealousy. But the details of your relationships are none of her concern, just as her love life is none of yours, unless she is asking for your advice.

8. How will our lifestyle influence the love lives of our children?

It will of course have an influence of some sort, but it's difficult to predict in what way, just as it's difficult to know how your emotional choices were influenced by those of your parents. Your love life alone will not influence your children, but rather your general way of being will. If you are evidently happy, then you will pass on this *joie de vivre*. If you are strict as they're growing up, while still allowing them their independence—the driving force of polyamory—then this combination of love, boundaries, and freedom will nourish their self-confidence. If they see that you are passionate about your work without being a work addict, they will understand that we come into our own when we do things because we enjoy them rather than need them. If they discover, little by little, that you yourselves are able to love more than one person without negative consequences, then they will free themselves from the myth of Prince Charming and his one princess, while still believing in love. Poly men and women who are plagued with guilt, on the other hand, who are so focused on their love lives that they don't pay enough attention to their children, or who choose polyamory out of spite, revenge, or boredom, will pass on these negative values to their children. This doesn't necessarily mean that their children will be doomed to a future of failed relationships, though; resilience, the ability to overcome challenges and to take positive lessons from them, may help these children, and it is also worth noting that children are capable of finding role models outside of the family unit. Given, however, that every human being is different, it is highly likely that each of your children will grow up with a different interpretation of their life experiences and potential traumas. There is no such thing as the perfect parent, and this is a fortunate thing. Given that parental mistakes affect children, imagine the case of a child with perfect parents who, when he reaches the age of rebellion, finds nothing he can reject in his adolescence and is therefore paralyzed by perfection!

Taking the Plunge

To paraphrase Simone de Beauvoir, one is not born poly, one becomes it. It is quite within the realm of possibility that, in the decades to come, we will see men and women entering relationships that they will immediately categorize as polyamorous, but, for the moment, this step is usually taken after an event that causes both parties to reflect upon their emotional commitments and the way they wish to live their lives.

More often than not, these triggers come in the form of a third person or an existential crisis. The partner who meets and falls in love with this third person suddenly realizes that it is possible for someone outside of his relationship to awaken desires and feelings within him, something which is widely known but that most continue to deny. This is a kick in the teeth for the myth that for each person there is one single other half just waiting to complete them. The person then thinks, "There are two people on this planet that I could fall in love with? Well then, why not three, or four, or more?" If the concept of "the woman/man of my life" is an illusion, then why sequester ourselves within the walls of monogamy?

If it were this easy to take the plunge, however, polyamory would be a worldwide romantic model! For me, polyamory came quite naturally early on, and I attribute this to my first heartbreak at the age of fourteen, when I stopped believing in Prince Charming. Myths are pretty tough-skinned, though, and, in an attempt to keep the myth of "one love" alive, people who fall in love with a second person will convince themselves that they must, by consequence, no longer love their present partner and that they should leave him or her. That is not something that is easy to do . . . especially if there is no real reason, outside of the fact that there is somebody else. There are several possible outcomes to this common dilemma: adultery, with its small secrets and big risks; separation from the lover in order to save the couple; separation from the partner in order to form a new couple with the lover, which could in turn end in separation, and so on and so forth; discussion with one's partner as to how wrong it would really be to live together happily, to feel good individually, while broadening romantic possibilities. Polyamory is born from this kind of dialogue, but there is one major hurdle. The balance between poly partners, as we have seen, is grounded in equality. During this initial stage, equality as we understand it is not really being respected, considering that the subject is brought to the table by the one who has fallen in love elsewhere. The other partner asked for none of it and, in most cases, is taken completely by surprise. A power struggle ensues wherein that partner feels betrayed and dragged down a path that he or she had not even imagined and is resistant, not because he or she is hostile toward polyamory as a concept, but because of the need to regain a certain level of control over the future. As for the other partner, the one who broached the idea of trying this different way of life, it is too late to backtrack without feeling frustrated or like she has given into her partner's jealousy.[24] This would be a form of self denial. A substantial shift in each perspective must occur until the point at which they both realize, accept, and then relish in the idea that two people who love each other have much better things to do than to try to get the upper hand over the other. Only then can the dialogue really begin. A working agreement has been reached, albeit with a set of training wheels to be slowly removed over time as the now poly partners discover that their new life is so natural and joyful that they forget the old one, much as we overcome fear. Fear sticks around in our memory for a while, but we usually find, after some time, that we can barely recall what it was that we were so afraid of.

Existential crises can arise after several years of living together and can just as easily crop up in a long-term relationship that has been, thus far, problem-free. What's changed? Nothing. Apart from, perhaps, a feeling of chronic dissatisfaction that is hard to deal with when

_____

24 These mechanisms are identical when the male/female roles in this equation are reversed.

there is nothing concrete on which to pin the blame. "In a matter of a few years," a young woman told me, "I got married, had a baby, started a business, made a decent amount of money, and bought a house. All this before I was thirty. But then at thirty, I asked myself if I had really chosen this path or if I had been pushed along it without thinking as a result of my upbringing and surroundings. I started dreaming of meeting other people who had nothing to do with our relationship, of traveling on my own, of taking up artistic interests; in other words, freedom. I visited an internet forum where people were talking about love with enthusiasm. I realized that that was what I needed. And then I met a man who understood exactly how I was feeling. . . ."

A midlife crisis can also sometimes act as a trigger: everything can be going just fine but, despite continuing feelings of love, you find yourselves increasingly unmotivated in the evenings, you go to bed earlier and earlier, you feel that nothing exciting is going to happen in the future, you hang desire at half-mast. "The routine" becomes the scapegoat, but, contrary to common belief, it is not routine that leads to dissatisfaction, but rather dissatisfaction that gives the impression of routine. When you're genuinely happy, then your habits—morning coffee, hot shower, flowers on a Sunday—do not seem routine but rather a kind of happy ritual. The same goes for making love. Feelings of boredom and routine are a manifestation of personal problems, difficulty relating to people, or existential anxiety, which leads us to question the choices we made in the past and those that may come in the future. Some couples, who have reached

the point of serenity often found in long-lasting relationships, decide to give polyamory a try in order to open
new doors to their existence, behind which they discover new people and previously unknown sides of their
own personality and sexuality. Many couples have experienced the occasional period of conjugal conflict or
breakup. They embrace polyamory with a desire to avoid
these unnecessary arguments, and a yearning to discover
that life can still be full of surprises. With their children
grown up and their professional hurdles cleared, they
begin this stage of maturity with the knowledge that the
plans they once made have been completed, and that
they can finally think of themselves. Taking the plunge
into polyamory may be psychologically easier for them
than for younger couples, who are still anxious about everything they have to prove. On the flip side of the coin,
it may take an older couple some time to feel comfortable with sex if they have never practiced it outside of
their relationship, and this feeling can be compounded
by the fact that their bodies no longer have all of the
qualities of youth to give them the assurance they need.

QUESTIONS

**1. Your book convinced me of the validity of polyamory,
but I'm not sure how to take the plunge.**

You don't know how to take the plunge . . . but you
just did! The hardest part is to understand that polyamory is a coherent, worthwhile romantic option, a perspective that was probably not part of your upbringing. Being
convinced by polyamory doesn't mean you have to jump

on the first person who comes along, but it does mean that you should allow yourself to love at a moment that you so desire. When this happens, you will get started quite naturally. But remember to find out what your partner thinks about it first!

2. I took the plunge. I found that it's actually very easy to have a lover, but I'm a little afraid: Given that it's so easy, won't I be tempted to sleep with everybody I meet?

Some people, as they begin their path of polyamory, feel the need to gorge themselves on love and seduction, so intoxicating is its simplicity that they can't believe they lived without it for so long. However, polyamory favors sustainable, emotional bonding, and so, soon enough, the time comes to separate the people you want to see again from those one-off or occasional dalliances. Being afraid of sleeping with everybody is a sure sign that you don't really want to. If that's the case, then don't do it, even though, as you say, it is rather easy.

3. I found myself in an unexpected situation with a woman and didn't want to let her slip away, so I took the plunge. Now I realize that it may not have been a one-off and I can't stand the idea of lying to my partner. I would like to talk her into polyamory too, but how can I bring it up without seeming like I'm presenting her with a *fait accompli*?

If you tell her what happened in order to convince her that polyamory is the right way for both of you to go, then you are presenting her with a fait accompli, but you're not lying to her. If you talk to her about polyamory in a more hypothetical manner—for example, if you tell her that you found a website on the subject, or that you read *To Love Several Men*—then you're lying by omission but are not presenting her with a fait accompli. Basically, you can't have it both ways, but does it really matter? You must choose the option that will allow you and your partner to discuss things rationally. It is not outside the realms of possibility, as we've seen, that your partner will respond that she has been thinking about polyamory without daring to talk to you about it, or that she has even had an affair herself that led her to feel this way!

4. Is it better to open up our relationship early on, or to wait until we start to get bored with our routine?

Polyamory can be a quick-fix remedy for conjugal boredom, but it will only stimulate a lagging libido in the short term, by momentarily reviving the inner narcissist. To make such a decision based on boredom, on a need to feel good about oneself, but not on desire, is an exercise in futility. The ideal thing to do is to discuss polyamory from the get-go, just as others express their needs for sexual exclusivity and even draw up prenuptial agreements. Unfortunately, this way of thinking is still a long way off. One day, however, when poly men and women are strong enough in numbers, polyamory will be seen as a realistic choice, based on the idea that it is natural to love and desire more than one person, and that plural love need not detract from any single one. Seen in this light, it will become a wondrous reality that anybody can adopt at as early a stage as possible, even before becoming part of a couple.

5. I have only ever slept with my partner. How do I make love to another man without seeming clumsy and foolish?

What a fine example of the way in which magazines and books make women feel that they must be experienced and technically apt in order to be good at making love! The essential factor is desire, which makes even the smallest caress feel like heaven. Practicing four hundred different sexual positions with a partner you don't desire is, at best, boring, and at worst, repulsive. Rest assured: When you find a man that you really desire, you won't be asking yourself if you're doing it well or not; it'll all come naturally.

Taking Each Day as It Comes

"Nothing is created or lost; it is merely transformed." Lavoisier's edict is in keeping with the philosophy of poly men and women, whose goal is not to set things in stone but to follow their natural evolution. This impermanence forces us to learn how to constantly adapt to change. In the time it has taken me to write these lines, dozens of events have taken place and changed the face of the earth as we know it, and this perpetual instability is a source of anxiety for many people. Stress, according to Hans Selye, a Canadian endocrinologist who studied its biological consequences, stems from the inability to adapt to changes, especially when they occur repeatedly and when people feel that they have no means of counter attack. Hence the powerful temptation to protect oneself by building a stable, concrete world, without surprises. In the letters I receive, I see the following phrases over and over again: "Are you sure that . . . ," "Can you promise me that . . . ," "Will I be safe if . . . ," and this despite the proof that nothing is set in stone in a field as volatile as love. Rather than disputing this proof, poly men and women accept the changeable nature of their situations, but also the permanent right to individuality.

More concretely, they do not force their relationships to be perpetually as they were at the beginning, and do not fight the waves of emotion and desire that inevitably occur at some time or another. They are smart enough to realize that you can't stop a river from flowing; you can merely change its course. On the other hand, they also know that not all situations are subject to this inevitable change: understanding that things could change in one sense, and then change back to where they were originally, they do not tend to split up over minor upsets. Polyamory allows time the slack it needs, knowing that it is the best remedy for both conflict and heartbreak. If they feel apprehensive about something, they realize that the feeling stems as much from the way in which they interpret the situation as it does from its objective reality. We are reminded of this subjectivity in our more mundane daily activities. For example, in a good mood, you may be whistling as you take the wheel, enjoying the scenery as you drive, smiling at the trees as they change color, relaxing at every red light. The next day, however, you dig your nails into the steering wheel without even glancing at the trees, grumbling because bad luck has it that you are getting stuck at all the red lights! It is not the situation that has changed, but your mood.

To be aware of the changeable nature of things, of situations, and of one's own moods, allows one to develop a sense of humor and an ability to distance oneself, if need be, in order to live a plural love life in the joyous, fulfilling manner it deserves to be lived. These qualities also allow poly men and women to deal with life's other worries, which is why outside observers often see them as carefree. They do not deny problems but have learned, rather, to dodge them for the time being, allowing time for the situation to improve instead of knocking their heads against a brick wall.

QUESTIONS

1. I am no longer "the one" for my partner, so how can I be sure that he really loves me?

You can never be absolutely sure of love; any woman whose husband leaves her after twenty years of monogamous marriage will tell you that.[25] Everything was going fine, she felt emotionally secure, and then, in a matter of minutes, her world was turned upside-down with her husband's announcement that he had fallen for someone else and was leaving. This separation is even more painful because this woman, as many others like her, had put everything into the existence of this love. But love is not a deal we make, nor is it an obligation: "You have to love me because I love you!" There is rarely an objective reason for falling in love, and the same goes for no longer loving somebody. The partner who

---

25 Françoise Chandernagor, *La Première Épouse* (*The First Wife*)— Gallimard, 1998.

continues to love can simply not understand what she has done to deserve the split. But the answer is simple: nothing. Heartbreak is so hard to bear because the ones who suffer have done nothing to deserve it, perhaps with the exception of couples who break up after years of incessant fighting. So in this way, being "the one" is not a guarantee of eternal love. Love is a feeling that knows no limits, not a cake that get smaller the more people there are to take a piece. Quite the opposite: Poly men and women show that it is possible to love exponentially. These people are, after all, in love with life itself and are open to spending time with whoever makes them happy. My experience, as well as that of many other poly men and women, is that an open, joyful, and playful relationship has a stronger chance of survival. Why leave somebody if you are happy with the things that you share, and have the added possibility of living other aspects of life in your own way? It is worth addding that even after they decide to separate their daily lives from each other, poly men and women often maintain emotional relationships with their exes, believing that just because some fundamental things have had to change, there is no need to close the door on the things that they still enjoy sharing.

2. My partner has just found out that I have been having polyamorous relationships and he wants to break up. I love him so much and want to share this way of loving with him—I just find it so much more gratifying and logical than jealousy!

Your partner is under enormous stress. You are asking him to make a huge shift in his way of thinking and being. Your love for him and his for you are not at issue here, but your situation is delicate and you're in the midst of a conjugal storm. It might be worth lowering the sails and sitting it out. Don't wear yourself out trying to explain things to him; he's not in a state where he will be receptive to it. This man needs you—go to him and allow him some time to renew his trust in you. Everything he believed in has changed, and he feels humiliated. Little by little, tell him about your desire. Not the desire you feel for such-and-such a man, but rather the desire for an open life, open to all sorts of possibilities. In other words, tell him about your philosophical ideals. Make it clear to him that you're convinced that therein lies your future happiness—with or without him, but preferably with. If he loves you and wants you to be happy as he says he does, then a real conversation can begin. If he insists that things return to the way they were before, then you have a choice: follow your desires and leave him, or stay with him and renounce them. At least the decision will be made with open eyes.

3. Will the desire I feel for my husband decrease as a result of physical passion with others?

Variations in levels of desire are inevitable. Even in a life of strict monogamy, you may feel less desire toward your husband at times, or perhaps none at all, just as he may one day desert you sexually. Desire is not linear: it does not start at the top only to inevitably dwindle. Rather, it is cyclical, and may disappear completely only to resurge at any given moment. It is an important aspect of love, but certainly not a vital one. Sex therapists can tell you that there are many couples who have little or no sex but who do not intend to separate because they enjoy many other things together. In polyamory, a temporary or long-term absence of desire is even less important, as fulfillment can come from other people, from lovers with whom you may not envisage sharing your life. A total loss of desire can also be a sign of unresolved conflict, health problems, or stress. By being aware of this instability, we stop using desire as an indicator of romantic feelings.

4. After years of polyamory, I am now living monogamously and am very happy about it. Was polyamory just a stopgap measure as I was waiting to find the perfect partner?

Tradition has always had it that men should sow their wild oats and experience love before "taking" a woman. Polyamory doesn't see the life of the couple as mutual appropriation, but rather as a way of love that is open to possibilities and that changes throughout one's lifetime. It's not a change in direction, but rather a change in situation, which doesn't erase the taste one has developed for polyamory. Being poly is part of your soul, even during single or monogamous periods. After all, it's a state of mind that implies being open to possibilities and not trapped inside dogma.

5. One of my lovers recently left me because he wants to settle down with someone and I'm not ready to share my life with him in this way. I understand his decision but miss him physically, despite my partner and other lovers. How can I overcome this heartbreak?

Polyamory doesn't protect you from heartbreak, but understanding its changeable nature allows you to cope with it better. Don't run from the feeling; accept it. It's painful, it upsets your stomach and eats away at your spirit, but you must deal with it on your own, or better, with a close friend. Remind yourself every day that you are going through a difficult, but temporary, period. Nothing is certain in life, except death. Your pain may seem never-ending, but it will eventually fade little by little. Perhaps tomorrow, another man will awaken that same level of desire in you. Perhaps your lover, having found a partner, will return to you to pick back up where you left off. Or you may become close friends, the memory of your shared feelings feeding that connection. Poly men and women don't deny that heartbreak exists, but know from experience that it eventually fades away and that plural love has the ability to resurge when we least expect it and to take surprising turns. Having such faith in life's surprises and an ability to take distance without feeling sorry for oneself means that heartbreak is a little easier to bear.

6. The way that you describe it, polyamory is a constant work in progress as you learn to adapt to situations that others would find unbearable. Does it really bring enough happiness to justify these efforts?

I've been poly for a long time, I wouldn't change it for the world, and if I had to start all over again, I would do things the same way. In this capacity, it is hard for me to answer in the negative! Efforts and hurdles are an integral part of successful polyamory because this lifestyle, which is constantly evolving, guards against the dreaded routine of the couple. It involves constant examination of the conditioning that we have been subjected to during our lives, and is therefore intellectually stimulating. It is certainly difficult to embark on polyamory without at least a little self-confidence and inner strength. But, by way of compensation, overcoming hurdles and experiencing those comical, or even surreal, events that dot the lives of poly men and women increase this strength as well as the ability to take a step back; two very useful things in the real world.[26] That which does not kill you only makes you stronger. Polyamory is starting to sound a little like Nietzscheism! Don't forget how great it is to love and be loved by men who will be with you for decades, will leave, and will come back to you, giving "impermanence" a delicious taste of eternity.

---

26 I was at a dinner recently where a woman was telling us about her and her husband's extra-marital affairs. The woman sitting next to her gave her a signal, and then announced to the rest of us, "I am one of her husband's lovers!"

Love and Laughter

L ove does not always equal fun. The melodrama of jealousy, the tragedy of breakups, the nostalgia for lost happiness . . . humans take their heartbreak very seriously. And so many refuse to take the wise advice of this comic: "In six months you'll have forgotten about it, so why not start now?"

Polyamorists are not necessarily humorists by nature, but they certainly become more so as time goes on and they realize that they must keep enough distance to be able to deal with unexpected situations safely, situations that may even make them laugh a few months down the line. Imagine the following scenarios: at your birthday party you find out that two of your best friends have started relationships with two of your lovers; you end up consoling one of your husband's lovers, who is beside herself with grief because he refuses to leave you for her; you find yourself trying to reassure a woman that her lover doesn't necessarily require erotic prowess, while at the same time slipping in a few hints as to the rudiments of male pleasure. These are but a few examples to show how rife with funny situations polyamory can be! Poly men and women, therefore, learn to identify the game behind every romantic connection, much like a staged fight that shouldn't be taken too seriously. They enjoy seducing and love to love, all the while remaining aware of the gap between the reality of feelings and the imagination of play.

A sense of playfulness helps to bring sex back down to earth by removing the high stakes that endanger it. This playful love can clear the way for poly relationships, where, much like the "let's pretend" of children's games, the imagination has free reign. To dramatize love a little is to give rightful credit to courting, flirting, and the little magical surprises that a person prepares for the one(s) they love. Enjoying erotic moments outside of the bedroom helps to add spice to life!

QUESTIONS

1. Doesn't "play," in the lighthearted, theatrical sense of the word, imply that you are just acting with your lovers and that you don't really love them?

Not at all! In the lighthearted sense of the word, playfulness means that love—be it marital or not—can be taken lightly sometimes, and is interpreted as a pleasure rather than a chore. Poly men and women enjoy making love, they laugh, they woo each other, they act the fool in ways that allow for both boldness and tenderness, and this playfulness helps keep their romances alive. As for the theatrical sense of the word, they enjoy acting, adore organizing magical evenings, slip into character, and invite their lovers to join them onstage and play along as they explore each other's fantasies. As opposed to swingers, however, who don't usually pursue relationships after an evening of sexual play, poly men and women carry their attentiveness to lovers into their "real" lives as well.

2. How can I keep my relationships casual but deep at the same time? I'm just not satisfied by these purely sexual affairs.

Paradoxically, casualness does not exclude depth, while superficial relationships can weigh on you in the long term. The purely sexual stage doesn't last long, though, as it is inevitable that two people who share pleasure will eventually develop more intimate bonds. That's where the poly arts of lightheartedness and laughter come into play: when feelings get complicated, poly men and women don't make a scene, but go with the flow with a smile on their lips. They never lose sight of the fact that loving someone is not the same as signing a contract for X number of years of exclusivity, nor does it require that they sever other romantic ties. To those in strictly monogamous relationships, or even theoretically polyamorous ones, this behavior is inconceivable. It's the kind of situation one could never imagine being in until it actually happens, but once it does, it seems like the most natural thing in the world.

3. How do I hang on to my playful side? As soon as I fall in love—which is quite often—I start to take myself so seriously!

It's hard for you to make love to someone you're not in love with, and what's wrong with that? You're not fifteen years old anymore, and you know the routine by now. You fall in love, convinced that you've met the "man of your life," but after a while, that love moves over to make room for another, and that one for yet another, each one as convincingly definitive in your mind. You'll hang on to your playful side when you see things clearly enough to conduct your relationships in the manner that children play games: with sincerity and conviction, but never losing sight of the fact that it's still a game. If you are overcome by passion and dream of leaving everything behind to be with the lover of the hour, then keep seeing him, but take your time before making any big decisions. With a little hindsight, you'll be able to tell whether your feelings were a result of love or a hormonal rush.

4. Isn't love more worthwhile when it's difficult, even impossible, rather than being one big game?

The tragedy of love sets the framework for the majority of novels and movies and has infiltrated our collective conscience. Why should misfortune be more worthwhile than fun and games? Polyamory, with its twists and turns, provides as much suspense as any tragedy, but allows for a little more fun along the way. An attraction to complicated relationships can be a dangerous thing. Many women lock themselves into the role of tragic lover with men they will never fully have because they are so content in their situation: they live the stuff of novels when they're with him, and spend the rest of the time feeling like a heroine in the grip of a dramatic affair. They cleanse themselves of the guilt of sexual desire by punishing themselves for the joy they experience but find impossible to accept. In all likelihood, if their lovers proposed to them, they would be completely thrown off guard, their whole framework crumbling around them. Neurosis of the heart, like any other neurosis, has its uses.

5. What is it about the art of playfulness that so many poly men and women have perfected? Whether with their partner or their lovers, poly men and women create intimate bonds without becoming completely attached. The intimacy they foster allows them to let loose in each other's presence, and this feeling of security is essential in any sexual play. Attachment, a source of dependency, is underlined by the fear of letting people down or dissatisfying them, feelings which shut the door on spontaneity. Whether the intimate relationship turns out to be a fiasco or a delight, the intimacy stays the same, interwoven with feeling and closeness. Sex in polyamorous relationships can sometimes be less dramatic, but it is certainly not sterilized, as is the case for swingers, who have sex with near strangers, without involving feelings.

Freedom

The idea of "freedom" has a tendency to frighten people and push them toward the more reassuring concept of "security." It is, however, perfectly possible for the two to coexist, when those who are free set their own boundaries in such a way as to enjoy risk-taking without complete recklessness. While freedom is certainly not the enemy of security, it is the antonym of the type of security that controls risks by enforcing codes of conduct, to the detriment of free will and individual trust. We live in a security-obsessed world, where more and more laws dictate, down to the most minute detail, how we should live our lives. Religious doctrine establishes prayer rituals, which is one thing, but also rules regarding food consumption, personal hygiene, and matters of sexuality and contraception. Those who do not practice religion are also seeing an increase in laws dictating how they should eat, drink, smoke, and make love. It is hard to turn on a TV without hearing about the importance of protecting ourselves against risks: from aggressive dogs to snowstorms, thugs, power lines, fairground rides, and swine flu. Not an object is sold these days that does not contain an extensive list of user precautions, often bordering on the absurd.[27] In short, risks and surprises are warded off by a generation of decision-making baby boomers, the first to have grown up without war and with a vastly reduced infant mortality rate, thanks to the progress of pre-natal medicine. They grew up believing they were invincible, but now discover with horror that nothing will save them from growing old and dying. A little reflection and work on the thought systems that gave rise to these problems would be quite enough to reassure them, but instead they pass their horror on to their children, who are brought up to believe that the survival of the planet and of humanity is in peril, that their jobs are at risk and their futures bleak.

Against this sensitive background, polyamory, with the trust, responsibility, and life-changing possibilities that it advocates, sticks out like a sore thumb. It is a form of freedom, however, that does know its boundaries. It trusts in the intelligence and wisdom of man and his ability to set his own limits and to respect his commitments. Poly men and women live their lives as they deem suitable, taking shortcuts at times but never underestimating the risks and never playing the hero.

---

27 "This Superman cape is only a toy and will not allow the consumer to fly," for example.

This responsible form of freedom teaches them to run from decisions that are imposed on them against their will, and to free themselves from the judgment of others, regardless of whether that judgment is passed in admiration or hostility.

QUESTIONS

1. Love is a bond that joins people together. Isn't that incompatible with this idea of freedom?

Romantic freedom doesn't give you free reign to do whatever you please. Poly men and women listen to the needs of the people they love because the bond they have formed is very important to them. It is precisely because these bonds are so important that they consider it unfair to be forced to leave somebody in order to have the right to love elsewhere. In the end, they are more faithful than people whose lives have consisted of successive monogamous relationships, where memories of previous ones are erased and treated as if they had never taken place. Bonds in polyamory are based on free consent and are not dictated by any kind of law or standard.

2. How can I make men understand that being poly doesn't mean that I want to jump on everything that moves?

They'll figure it out soon enough when you reject their advances, especially if, to their inevitable statement, "But I thought you were a free woman?" you respond, "Freedom is about saying no when I don't feel like it."

3. Is it ok if I approach men that I find attractive?

Of course, as long as you accept that you may get a few surprised looks. It's easier to meet people at a friend's house, on vacation, at work, or through other activities that involve a lot of socializing. Men will be delighted to chat with you and pleased at your interest in them. If you approach people on the street, on the other hand, you may catch them off guard, given that the idea of a woman making the first move or suggesting something as minor as having a coffee together is still quite alien to most men. But if you're game and are not afraid of failure, then why not? Men have been asking women out for centuries and manage to survive rejection. This hasn't stopped them from maintaining their dominating position in society! It is better, however, if you know a little about the male race, as this will help you to spot the macho, the conqueror, the pervert, or the easily shocked, who may not know how to take your advances. Once you've figured out which ones to avoid, the others will be happy to feel desired. It probably doesn't happen to them all that often!

4. My partner won't accept polyamory, but spends his time meeting women in internet chat rooms. How can we both enjoy our respective freedom?

Virtual relationships allow us to introduce the best side of ourselves with our most flattering photos and embellished details of our lives. It's even possible to invent a whole new personality. Also, the knowledge that you can pull the plug on it at any given moment allows for a feeling of supreme power. Many people are happy with this and never want to meet the person with whom they are conducting a wild cyber affair. Virtual flirting is different from its real life counterpart but comes from the same motivation: to stimulate the libido and reassure oneself of one's ability to seduce. It's an exercise in narcissism as opposed to polyamory, which is an exercise in exploration. It's not that strange that you and your partner are on different wavelengths, and if you're able to discuss things and agree on a certain level of respective romantic freedom, then it is quite possible to compromise and live in keeping with your individual desires.

5. After a few drinks too many, I stupidly told my boss that I was poly. Since then he's been hounding me to be his lover, but I just don't want to. How can I turn him down without risking my job?

If ignoring his advances is not having the desired effect, then it's time to take the bull by the horns. Explain to him that polyamory is about freedom, in particular the freedom to say no, and that, in addition, you don't like to mix business with pleasure. If he continues and threatens you with reprisal, start collecting his letters and emails or even record his phone calls, and then tell him that you'll file a complaint if he doesn't leave you alone. Sexual harassment is a punishable crime.

6. How can I explain to my future husband that I'm poly and that I'd like to keep this freedom after we marry?

Exactly like that. Explain to him that you agreed to get married because of how much you love him, but that you've learned over the years that your happiness is greater when nourished by freedom and variety. Let him consider this new idea for a while, as well as the fact that he too would be able to love other women, and don't hesitate to talk about it together. Push the wedding back a little if you need to, but make sure it takes place on solid ground. Don't forget to point out that being poly doesn't mean you'll be sleeping around all the time! In all likelihood, at the beginning of your marriage you'll be so engrossed in each other that you'll be more or less monogamous.

7. Does polyamory sometimes take freedom a bit too far?

Who can say what "too far" means? There are just two instances where you can be said to have overstepped the mark: firstly, if you stop being considerate of those you love, and secondly, if your romantic behavior is no longer dictated by desire but by force. Remember, too, that romantic freedom is not just about sex, but also tenderness, caresses, and even just words. It's not like it is on some internet sites where you first select a sexual practice (fellatio, S&M, etc.), as if you were shopping for a camera, and then look for the partner who will help fulfill that fantasy. There is no consideration in those cases for the individuals, who all become one, anyway, after completion of the desired act. Polyamory works in quite the opposite way: you meet people first, and then you decide what you'd like to do together.

Passion

When people fall in love, they would do well to remember that the word "passion" comes from a Latin verb which means "to suffer." The passion of Christ did not have a whole lot to do with pleasure, given that it was a crucifixion! But this has not stopped romantic passion—and the insanity, crime, and death that can follow as a consequence—from fascinating many and from being interpreted as a sign of Love, with a capital L. Poly men and women are not exempt from this, but they are less likely to fall victim to a passion that years of experience has taught them to understand as vain and often fleeting, despite its promises of eternity. They enjoy it as a theatrical episode in their love lives and are less susceptible to dependency than they would be if that passion were their sole fixation.

QUESTIONS

1. Do people choose polyamory because they're afraid of passion?

Polyamory does seem at first to shy away from passion because, even though it is quite possible to love more than one person at a time, simultaneous passionate relationships are hard to maintain. However, people don't decide to love more than one person as a way of avoiding passion, but rather out of a curiosity about others and a desire to find out more about themselves. Poly men and women may go through wildly passionate stages in their relationships, but their consciousness of the evolving nature of love and their sense of humor allow them to play with fire without getting burned.

2. Can we really be in control of our relationships if passion, as you have pointed out, is a hormonal impulse that defies reason?

It's not a question of running your love life like you run a business, nor is it about restraining desire. On the other hand, it is important to remind ourselves of the biological nature of passion and its ability to make us "crazy" for somebody. It is unwise to make important decisions (breakups, pregnancy, suicide) under the influence of passion, as it can be hard to distinguish between the "crazy" and the real-life aspects of these impulses. Enjoy passion while it lasts, but don't let it break you. If you don't feel you can handle it, get out of the relationship. In the early stages of passion, it is still possible to escape if things seem to be getting out of control. After those first stages, things can get a little tricky.

3. A lover whom I simply adore has been begging me for three years to get divorced and move in with him. I thought about it for a long time and when I finally decided to go for it, he said he'd changed his mind and wanted to stay with his wife. I was very hurt by this about-face, and we broke up. I feel crushed: he's the only person that's ever treated me like this. Other lovers, whom I've been less passionate about, have always been wonderful to me.

In all likelihood, his persistent requests were driven by his desire to test the power he held over you, by asking you to do something drastic, such as divorce your husband. The romantic freedom you enjoy as a poly woman bothered him and made him jealous, so he was trying to throw you off balance. In the end, the passion you shared stemmed from a dynamic of domination rather than true love, but this doesn't mean that the moments you shared are any less valuable. Give your wounds some time to heal. You're lucky that you have other lovers around to comfort you, even if they'll never take this man's place. Why did you fall head over heels for him and not the others? Now is as good a time as any to ask yourself what could have led you to this painful situation, and what intimate need this passion provided for.

4. For the first time in my life, I feel I am physically addicted to a lover whom I'm actually not even in love with. In between dates, it's like I'm in withdrawal—it's not love, it's a drug!

Sexual pleasure releases endorphins, which are often dubbed "natural morphine." Comparing it to a drug is not far off the mark. Some people get consumed by these kinds of relationships, which, for them, don't bring love, but trouble and destruction. Others find it stimulating and enjoy pushing their partners' limits in dominant/submissive role play, where the roles are interchangeable. Your task is to decide whether this sexual dependence is having a positive or negative effect on you. If it's negative, then run away. Polyamory should enhance your love of life, not distort it.

Sex

If polyamory had nothing to do with sex, then there wouldn't be nearly as many problems associated with it as there are, except for couples in which one partner is compulsively jealous and doesn't like the other to enjoy a private life or platonic friendships outside of the relationship. Sex, however, does play a particularly important role in polyamory, but perhaps not the one that people automatically imagine. An American psychiatrist recently said that partner traders found that their nerves were calmed by making love more often than usual, and concluded: "They tend to turn to unhealthy cures for their problems, such as alcohol, drugs, and sex." An odd choice of grouping, just like this one: on television, sex is systematically linked to violence in the realm of movie ratings, as if it has been forgotten that sex is fundamentally based on emotions and not on violence.

The economy is more present in the media than sex, but we do not see people complaining about the negative effects of this, despite the fact that, in other areas of our lives, it is a greater cause of violence. On the other hand, the negative aspects of sex are constantly being discussed, and during these conversations we see prostitution rings and sex crimes thrown together under the same banner of shame as pornographic images, which may not be aesthetically pleasing to all, but are not deadly. I once appeared on a television show on the channel Europe 1, during which Matthiew Lindon, a journalist for the French newspaper *La Libération* pointed out that the media never talks about the happiness that results from sex, but focuses only on the guilt and criminality often associated with it. This is no accident. By presenting sex in a negative light, we attach a sense of anxiety to it, certainly the last thing needed, considering the extent to which sex is already weighted down by religious guilt. Even articles about sexual pleasure make it in to something complicated, detailing lists of techniques that imply an intimidating obligation to perform correctly, and relegate the issue of desire to second place.

In the context of all this, thinking of sex as a natural and unique way of connecting with other people is considered subversive. Not for moral reasons, given that it seems perfectly acceptable to boast about one's own sexual exploits and to gossip about politician and celebrity sex scandals, but rather because the concept of joyful pleasure, open to anybody, is in direct contrast with society's values. This way of thinking is subversive because it accepts that sex is not intrinsically harmful, and makes the link between romantic myths and the three major narcissistic blows dealt to the human race over the course of its history.

The first came from Copernicus: When he, along with Giordano Bruno and Galileo, announced that the earth was, in fact, a planet rotating around the sun, and not, as common belief then had it, the center of the universe, their discovery lead them to be judged and condemned for ruining man's desire to be the center of all. Then came Darwin, with an even harder kick in the teeth: the human race was not a product of God's Petri dish but rather descendant from unicellular organisms, primitive animals, and monkeys. Freud came along to offer a third blow by showing that man is not rational, does not make decisions freely, but is instead lead around by the nose and the genitals, directed by the unconscious, which by its very nature as such cannot be vanquished.

Dare I suggest that the reevaluation of the monogamous couple is a continuation of this kind of attack? Absolutely, given that the monogamous couple is a narcissistic construction wherein each partner wants to possess the other and feel assured that, in his partner's eyes, he is the one and only. At the risk of greatly reducing its size, he aims to become the center of that person's universe and to deny her the opportunity of meeting new people and of other activities that make up life itself. In so doing, he centers his existence around this concept: "We fell in love, we will be in love for ever, so please, shut the door on the things and people that could change you." The hidden impulses of desire are, needless to say, not permitted either: behind the familiar door of marital desire lies another door, which in turn may reveal another, more mysterious one, behind which may lie one's true animal self. Understanding these narcissistic stakes is the best way to understand why sex still frightens some people, and the ways in which polyamory allow us to deal with Copernican, Darwinian, and Freudian anxieties; in other words, reality.

QUESTIONS

1. What are the benefits of sex in a relationship that isn't headed toward the long term?

Sex is the richest communication method we have as humans, because it uses every one of our senses. In our daily lives, we are used to communicating using sight and language, sometimes touch, but rarely taste and smell. Making love creates an intimacy that is hard to find elsewhere. People tend to open up and confide in their lovers after sex, even if they have trouble expressing their feelings in the context of their daily lives. Sex brings pleasure, but is not without its risks, and underestimating its potential impact on the unconscious can be dangerous. And, even though they often coexist, sex is not the same as love or life commitment. It is quite possible to love having sex with someone with whom you have no wish to spend your daily life, and, the other way around, you may live happily with someone with whom sex takes second place. Polyamory allows us to see to that love, sex, and relationships are not as inseparable as we have been lead to believe.

2. What is the basis of a relationship if there is no promise of sexual fidelity?

This question makes it look as though sex were the standard gauge of love, more important than shared living, intellectual affinity, or tenderness. Yet, supposedly "faithful" people will fool around with strangers at swinger clubs or visit prostitutes, all the while telling themselves, "It doesn't matter; it's just sex." When we hear the expression, "There's nothing between us," we are supposed to interpret it as "nothing sexual," even if the protagonists concerned feel strongly for each other. In other words, the emphasis put on sexual fidelity is not a sign that sex is a necessary proof of love, but rather that there is an enormous amount of uneasiness still surrounding sex and desire. To answer your question more specifically, being in a couple consists of shared activities, mutual trust, joy in each other's company, and a meeting of the minds.

3. Is polyamory likely to lead me to try other things, like group sex or S&M? Should I set limits for myself?

When it comes to sex, anything is possible between consenting adults. If a lover tries to lead you down a path that you don't wish to follow, then refuse. There's one good way to figure out what you want: if you wake up the morning after with a sort of hangover, a mix of shame and disillusionment, then it probably wasn't right for you and you shouldn't pursue it further. If, however, you wake up with a smile still on your lips, then there's no problem, even if you have broken your barriers and tried something you never imagined possible.

4. Why does my husband share his fantasies with other women when I am extremely open and would love to share them with him?

Our fantasies are the most secret part of our being, the fine line between the conscious and unconscious. Some are so far removed from how we see ourselves— perhaps revealed in an erotic dream—that they can be shocking and even frightening. Add to that the fact that the couple is slippery ground and the stakes are high: power, money, children. It is not always the most desirable place to reveal this peculiar part of your unconscious. Also, some fantasies may simply not be suitable for sharing, because they would shock or offend the other person. For example, if a woman dreams of watching two men making love, but her husband, while not homophobic, is decidedly straight, then sharing this fantasy with him would be problematic, since asking him to fulfill it would be impossible. And of course, if he did do it out of love and a desire to please his wife, it would inevitably end in disaster.

It is also important to remember that fantasies are reliant on the chemistry between two individuals. The idea of his lover in a maid outfit may turn on a man who would find it ridiculous, or even sick, to see his wife dressed up in the same way.

There's one last possible explanation for your husband's preference for sharing his fantasies outside of the home: so many marriages these days end in divorce, and partners begin scrabbling around, looking for any dirt they can throw in order to win a larger settlement. It can be to share your fantasies with your wife, knowing in a corner of your mind that she may, five years down the line, claim in court that you're a pervert for tying her to the bedpost, or with your husband, who could later blame you for having group sex, even if it was he who suggested it at the time.

5. Why is it that I enjoy playing erotic games with my lovers, but would never dream of doing the same with my husband?

Perhaps your relationship with your husband is more about love than sex, which is particularly likely if you met when you were very young. Your libido with him has stayed at a stage when the two of you had sex because you were in love, and not because of a taste for eroticism. After years of meeting other people, you have explored your sensual side, but your relationship with your husband has kept its initial innocence. Another theory is that he sees you more as a wife and mother than a mistress, and this is hardly likely to inspire you to break out your most sensual self. Perhaps he made an offensive, macho comment about "horny" women, and this has put you off. Perhaps you can only really let yourself go when you maintain a certain emotional distance from someone, which would explain your increased comfort with lovers as opposed to your husband. You may fear that by adding this extra link—that of sexual attachment—you risk becoming too dependent on him. It may be that all of these are factors coexist, if for the most part in your unconscious.

6. Polyamory has liberated me sexually to such an extent that I've become obsessed with sex!

In the grips of new pleasures, we tend to think about sex more than usual, and perhaps more than is reasonable, but what a beautiful thing it is sometimes to be unreasonable! However, poly men and women actually tend to be less obsessive about sex than those who are frustrated due to monogamy. They don't visit as many porno sites and tell fewer dirty jokes for the simple reason that they are not deprived of anything. Sex is no longer a haunting, forbidden pleasure. They have sex when they feel like it and can make the time for it, but abstain if it's not a good time, safe in the knowledge that each period of romantic fasting is temporary and usually followed by a period of exquisite feasts. Nonetheless, a little sexual obsession, as long as it stays in the mind and doesn't bother anybody else, is no more dangerous than a passion for movies or stamp collecting.

7. This polyamory thing—doesn't it take up too much of your life? Now that I've reached an age where my "pants are peaceful," so to speak—being at an age where erections are not what they once were—I realize how much time I dedicated to sex in the past. Now I have time for other activities and find them to be just as satisfying!

The culprit here is not polyamory, but your libido! Studies suggest that young men, faithful or not, married or single, are not capable of going three minutes without thinking about sex. As we have seen, obsession is fuelled by frustration. Polyamory takes up too much space within the couple if those involved are so obsessed with living "outside the norm" that they allow their endeavors to dominate conversation. For this reason, among so many others, it will be better for all when poly-amory becomes more commonplace.

Conclusion . . . To Be Continued

In early 2003, I interviewed a scientist whose ground-breaking research, regularly published in the prestigious scientific revue *Nature* in the 1980s, had come under attack from the scientific community because it required a major shift in what are considered to be the accepted laws of biology. He complained about his peers' inability to move forward in their thinking, pointing out that accepting modern mathematics had not meant throwing out Euclidean geometry, and that refusing to question previous ways of thought would not allow humanity to evolve. "These days," he lamented, "we don't burn non-believers—we just cut their funding."

After our lunch, the conversation turned to my projects, and I told him about To Love Several Men, which had recently been published. To my great surprise, he flew in to a rage at the concept of polyamory, which was all the more surprising because I thought he seemed like quite the ladies' man! "You're talking about something that can't exist, it's simply impossible!" he blurted.

I told him about my personal experiences, as well as those of a good number of my readers, and reminded him that monogamy only applies to a small portion of humanity and is extremely rare in the animal kingdom (which includes us), but he was adamant. I singled out a few of his colleagues, known for leading double, or even triple, lives, and in response he snapped, "Well, of course it's possible for men, but not for women." His belief, to which he clung with quite frightening determination, was that women are only able to fall in love with men who can give them orgasms, and that once this has occurred, they are willing to give up anything—their husbands, even their children—for that man. "That's just how they're made: when a woman has an orgasm, she becomes dependent—it's biology. Your theory signifies the end of the family, even the end of civilization!" In his angry state, his manner of speaking became decidedly disrespectful. I countered that my "theory," as he called it, was based on many years of experience, and that, as in many poly relationships, there were children involved. Moreover, I told him, I never said that I was trying to replace monogamy with polyamory, but that I hoped that, in light of the growing number of failed marriages, I could show that there were other romantic possibilities out there. But he would not budge.

This man, shunned by his colleagues because they did not appreciate him calling their long-held convictions into question, was demonstrating the exact same attitude: point-blank refusal to think outside of the box and explore the unknown, a positively antiscientific mindset which, ten minutes earlier, he'd found so horrifying in other researchers. I understood, at that moment, just how difficult it is for even intelligent, well-educated, inquisitive beings such as scientists to think outside of their usual logic system. Especially when the new idea pulls the rug out from underneath something that they want to believe in—in this case, that men are strong and women are emotionally fragile.

November 2008: In preparing this book, I put out a call for testimonials. Along came Stephen, Sonia, and Andrew,[28] a classic trio: husband, wife, and lover. The simple version of the story is this: After six hectic years—marriage, baby, own business, own house—Sonia felt trapped in a life that was moving too quickly. Her weariness had affected her feelings of desire within her marriage, and her anxiety was even harder to bear because she felt that she had everything to be happy about and felt guilty for not being so. Existential angst: "What do I really want?" And then, what she really wanted entered the room like a breath of fresh air when she met a group of artist bloggers, their eyes wide open but feet still firmly on the ground. She quickly became involved in an intensely emotional, sexual relationship with Andrew, one of the group, but did not consider leaving Stephen for a second. He was her future, but she felt the need to explore other worlds, to feel free. "When I read your book," she told me, "I wasn't struck as much by your open sex

28 Their names have been changed.

life as I was by the story of your trip to Greece, alone, for two months. How lucky you were to be able to balance this with your marriage and children!" And then, the inevitable: Stephen accidentally found out about Sonia's affair. The usual ballet ensued, spinning from conflict ("Leave this man, now!"), to heartbreak, to lies, to sudden changes of heart. Stephen himself had been tempted in the past, but had never given in because he did not wish to be unfaithful to Sonia. I pointed out to him that it was perhaps not Sonia's desire for Andrew that was a shock for him but the infidelity, the lies, and the feeling that she had acted without talking to him first, with no consideration for their relationship. His ego had taken a beating, from which he was struggling to recover. He agreed and went so far as to say that once his wounds were healed, he might even be able to accept Sonia's relationship with Andrew, especially if it meant that he too could benefit from a new openness in their marriage.

Fast-forward to Stephen's final message, after I told him that the essential issue—more important than Sonia's affair with Andrew, which was on hold for a while—was the anxiety that had led Sonia to it in the first place. The two of them could not afford to neglect this aspect of their future together:

> We can't just get back together as things were before, because she would be heartbroken at the breakup of her relationship. There would be no fertile soil in which to re-grow our love for each other. I have come to understand Sonia's need to be free, and any attempt on my part to change her would be doomed from the start. Per-

sonally, I need to feel secure, to feel that my other half is devoted to me. But I am ready to find a compromise between my needs and Sonia's personality, both because I love her, and because I need to quell my anxiety. Today, I don't just consider my own needs, but also my wife's. At least this painful experience has taught me to do that. Finally, I don't want to feel that she's the one in control of our love life.

The events of the past two weeks seem to have helped Sonia think about what she really wants, which is a good thing. She has come to see that whatever happens must be in keeping with me as a person who, as you well know, is changing for the good of us both. With warm regards.

PS. It would be wonderful if we could meet again in a year to talk about all of this.

Several days later, I received a desperate letter from a man whose wife had fallen in love with another woman and was going to leave him, without a second thought for their children or the life they had built together. I explained to him that it would be next to impossible to talk to her while she was in this early stage of passion, as it would make her both blind and deaf to reason. "You must accept the passion she is experiencing," I told him, "which is more powerful than either of you. But ask her to postpone her decision for at least six months, if possible. This may allow you to communicate with each other and to find a compromise that will suit everybody involved."

Later, he sent me a copy of this letter, addressed to his wife:

I wanted you to stay with me tonight, but I under-stand that you needed to be with E. I have been looking at our photos: our family is so beautiful, we were so happy.

I ask you to please reconsider my offer. I don't want you to leave like this, I don't want you to break our family apart before you've had time to think about it. Take some time before you make your decision. We will have to change things around in order to continue to be a family, but it's not that hard. I love you, and to me, that means seeing that you are happy and fulfilled (emotionally and sexually), with me or with someone else, but still by my side. I believe that it's possible to love more than one person in more than one way—I know it's not the way things usually work, but that's life!

After everything we've built up and been through together, it must be worth a try. If it works, then great. But if it doesn't work, then we'll call it a day then. This new life might be difficult at first, but it will also be full of passion and pleasure, and the added bonus that it allows us to keep our family together, our children.

Think about it. For my part, I am ready to give it a go, to accept it openly and respect your wishes. Just the possibility is already calming me down, I won't be quite so sad as I climb into bed.

His note to me continued:

Please excuse the plagiarism, but your words [about acceptance and hope] were so helpful to me, and also to my wife, who had feared we would tear each other apart. Through your expressions I was able to communicate more clearly with her, to express my feelings more easily. I am quite a reserved person, and a combination of my difficulty in expressing myself and the hectic nature of our lives (work, worries, children, etc.) has created a distance between us, always pushing difficult conversations to the next day.

Since that letter, we have both been doing better. We are talking a lot; about us, her, them, the children, the immediate future. She seems to be very much in love with her girlfriend but I am hopeful (although not naïvely so) that we may be able to save our family.

She is, however, finding it difficult to understand my reaction. She's not sure how I am able to accept the situation, but she is happy about it, as she had feared things would get messy.

Even misfortune can have fortunate consequences. All this has forced me to reflect on our relationship, on our children, on life, and even a little bit on myself: what it is that I want and don't want out of life. We were always making plans, putting things off until the next weekend, etc. That was all a mistake. You must take what life has to offer and live in the moment.

I love this quote from the Dalai Lama: "Whether we are feeling happy or unhappy at any given moment often has very little to do with our absolute conditions but, rather, it is a function of how perceive our situation, how satisfied we are with what we have."

A few years ago, these two couples would have divorced in a cloud of violence and resentment. Today they are able to have a dialogue and to understand the thought each other's processes, no matter how far removed from their own. They talk of love and not possession.

If I have played even the smallest part in this, then I am truly happy.

The Etiquette of Polyamory

Polyamory will inevitably give rise to unforeseen situations, and the men and women involved must know how to deal with them in the heat of the moment. This guide is not exhaustive by any means, but it offers answers to some frequently asked questions.

1. Should we draw up a "dating schedule"?

The idea is that both partners have the same level of autonomy. Sharing "date days"—you on Tuesday, me on Thursday—is one practical solution, especially if you have small children. But this schedule should allow for a little flexibility. Your wife shouldn't feel that she has to force herself to go out on a day when she doesn't feel like it, just because it's "her day." If a lover asks her to go out on a Wednesday, but her day is Tuesday, then it's polite to accept a little bending of the rules. A schedule is reassuring at the beginning because it sets some limits

The Art and Etiquette of Polyamory

to the outside relationships and provides each partner with some sort of reference point, and it helps to know in advance if your partner won't be there on this day or that. But bit by bit, you will slip into a pattern and the schedule will no longer be necessary. Poly men and women learn quickly to split their time between their family and private lives, and to adapt the initial rules accordingly. For example: you continue to go out on Tuesdays and Thursdays while your husband isn't really seeing anybody at that moment. If he is happy with that and takes the opportunity to see his friends or just hang out at home, then there isn't a problem. If it is difficult for him, then it is his responsibility to express that to you so you can work together to find a solution that suits everybody. Polyamory is a conversation where each person says how he/she feels, without trying to come out on top. This is a relatively new way of structuring a couple, which is traditionally rife with power struggles.

2. How do I find the time to date more than one person when I am so busy?

Time has its limits, and so to find enough of it for your love life, you must sift through and pick out what is essential and what is secondary within your activities. In reality, this question no longer applies when desire comes into play: lovers will always manage to find time for one another! Exceptions to that, of course, would be while taking care of a newborn child, after illness, or during particularly stressful times at work. Politicians, corporate tycoons, and celebrities are notorious for leading plural love lives, despite the nature of their rather demanding professions. Why is this not the case for everybody else? Why do so many people put love in second place, prioritizing other activities, including cleaning and even watching television? Because they dare not do otherwise and feel guilty for thinking of themselves. They tell themselves that pleasure is a privilege they do not deserve, but if it were free and uncomplicated, then it would be accessible to all.

3. At first, the deal was that each of us could go out one night a week, until 2 a.m. Soon we added the option of staying out overnight, and now my partner wants to spend the weekend with her lover. I agreed to this on the condition that I would be allowed to do the same thing. Shouldn't the only real rule be to make decisions together and to keep things on an equal footing?

Rules are broken when actions no longer represent mutual agreement, just as laws need a majority vote to be passed. It is important not to impose your view on your partner, who will then find him or herself in a position of constantly trying to break the rules. The best thing to do is to decide upon an initial modus vivendi and adjust it as you become more sure of yourselves and your choices. You will eventually reach a point at which you do not feel it necessary to establish rules because they now come naturally. Remember, though, that this does not mean that you don't have a right to be upset if you think your partner has overstepped the mark.

4. Once we've agreed on polyamory, do I have to tell my partner every time I'm dating someone new, or is

it enough to just say, "I'm going out tonight," without specifying whether it is with a friend, a cousin, or a lover?

Nothing is set in stone. The rules result from partner agreements, which are constantly updated. At the start, many women, conditioned to believe in male "unfaithfulness impulses," are inclined to say, "Do what you want, just don't tell me about it." Men, reluctant to lose control of their partner and fascinated by the most recent manifestations of her libido, are likely to use the idea of "transparency" as a cover-up for wanting to know everything she does. As time goes on, those involved become more self-assured and are often satisfied with knowing that their partner has someone else, without needing all of the details. They tell each other that they're going out, at what time they will return, and, if need be— although this is not an obligation—with whom. Future conversations will be more focused on the philosophy of polyamory, and then after a while, they won't even feel the need to talk about it very much at all.

5. Under the banner of independence, my partner spends less and less time at home, and spends more time with his lover than with me, including weekends and vacations. Is this acceptable?

It's acceptable as long as you are not suffering as a result. If, however, this neglect is hurting you, then there is no reason for you to put up with it. Freedom and independence are not excuses to do whatever you want. Respecting your partner's freedom shouldn't mean letting him hurt you in the process. Talk to him about it rationally, being careful not to throw accusations around.

And express your feelings as precisely as you can: "I feel a bit neglected," "I would like us to spend more time together," and so forth. It is important to identify where your anxiety is coming from. Is it a real desire to spend more time with him, or a feeling that you're losing him or the control that you previously had over the relationship? Is it actually heartache, manifesting itself through jealousy, or the fact that he is being inconsiderate? As for your partner, he must decide whether he is neglecting you because his inner narcissist is feeding off of this current stage of seduction, because he is testing his power over you by making you jealous, because his lover has asked him to "prove his love," or simply because he is in love with her, and less so with you. The reasons for his behavior are more important than the behavior itself, which could be temporary or, on the other hand, be a sign that things between you are coming to an end.

6. How should I deal with unforeseen problems, for example missing the last train and having to stay overnight with a lover?

You must call your partner immediately so she doesn't worry when you're not there in the morning. If it's too late to call, then at least send a text message that she will read first thing when she wakes up.

7. Should I leave some time in between dates?

Preferably, yes, but there are always exceptions. Tacking one evening of sex onto another could cause you to burn out or, on the other hand, become so dependent on pleasure that you need to "increase the dosage" in order to be satisfied. Sex can become an addiction, with all the symptoms of drug addiction: dependency, dissatisfaction, distancing oneself from others. In any case, the body needs to recharge from time to time!

8. My partner has a smitten lover who calls him at all hours of the night. How can I put a stop to this intrusion without jeopardizing my partner's freedom?

One partner's freedom should not invade the life of the other. Ask your partner to turn off his cell phone and put the answering machine on the house line after a certain time in the evening. If he refuses, then make him sleep somewhere else—he'll soon understand that he's going too far. If he accuses you of restricting his freedom, he's confusing freedom with free-for-all.

9. How should I respond to my partner's jealous lover who sends me hateful text messages simply because I'm the one he chooses to live with?

Tell your partner to intervene and stop this hateful behavior. If that's not enough, change your cell phone number. By the way, how did she get hold of it in the first place?

10. How can I explain to the wife of an old friend that I would like to have him to myself sometimes? He's the one I confide in, not her.

Close friendships are often hard for a partner to accept because they feel excluded. It is perfectly understandable that you would want to spend time alone with your friend, but it's his job to make his partner understand this and to come up with some sort of system whereby your meetings suit everyone involved.

11. My husband took one of his lovers to his parents' house for dinner. Now they assume that we have split up and have stopped inviting me! How can we sort out this misunderstanding?

Mixing your poly life and family life, especially with relatives who aren't necessarily open to the idea, is a huge mistake and demonstrates disrespect for you. There isn't much choice at this point but to tell them—and this is his job—that the mix-up is his fault and that he is sorry that his lack of etiquette has made you all suffer as a result. Of course, if you don't miss those dinners with the in-laws, then that step is unnecessary and would only upset them. The issue at stake here is how your resentment toward your partner—who has pushed you to the side—is going to affect your relationship.

12. We put our poly life on hold on weekends, which we save for family time. But what if one Saturday, a lover whom I don't see very often is in town for just one night? Am I allowed to depart from the usual rules in a case like this?

Anything is possible. Rules are made not to be broken, but to be adapted to unexpected situations. There is, therefore, nothing wrong with seeing your lover on a Saturday, as long as your partner is all right with it. However, if she's prepared a special dinner for your anniversary or some other special occasion that night, it goes without saying that you must say no to your lover.

13. I bumped into my boss when I was out with one of my lovers, and introduced her as my wife. Now my actual wife won't come to meet me at work and is angry that I "erased her" in an act of cowardice.

Poly men are more likely than women to get themselves in these impossible situations. In the same situation, your wife would probably have simply waved to her boss, introducing her lover by his first name only with such ease that her boss would have forgotten the whole thing by the time he turned the corner. What's done is done, and now you must apologize and try to regain your wife's trust. Why not take her along to your office holiday party and introduce her as your new partner? Given the current divorce rate, probably no one will even bat an eyelid!

14. My lover doesn't like meeting in hotels and invited me to his place, but it makes me uncomfortable to make love in the bed he shares with his wife.

The marital bed is a powerful symbol, but there are other options. Why not try the living room couch, the kitchen table, or his desk chair? Chances are you'll both find this extremely erotic and he will never look at his furniture in the same light again! Alternately, you could find a friend who doesn't mind lending you her apartment for a few hours.

15. How should I react to the rude comments I get for being seen as a sexually liberal woman?

There are a few options: 1) ignore them, and the men or women making these remarks will eventually give up; 2) make the commenters themselves out to be sex-obsessed and point out that your freedom comes hand in hand with a level of discretion, from which they could perhaps take an example; 3) go along with it and throw in a few details that are so obscene they will beg you to stop and never bring up your sex life again; 4) get them where it hurts and say similar things about them, preferably in front of their partners, to make them see how inappropriate and stupid such lewd behavior really is. The last two options are particularly effective!

16. How should I react to aggressive women who accuse me of trying to steal their husbands?

Poly women frighten some wives, who have it all backward given that the logic of polyamory is contrary to the logic of ownership. Humor is perhaps your best weapon in this case: it may not reassure all women, but at least it lightens the atmosphere and makes you feel a little better. Feel free to borrow a phrase from one of my articles: "I sometimes borrow married men, it's true, but I always give them back in good condition." Throwing this little joke out there allows you to set the record straight. You could also whisper in her ear that men are rarely raped and that, far from being victims, they are fully aware of their actions when they cross the line into adultery. Finish by expressing your constant shock that wives and partners are always convinced that other women want to steal their man, as if he were the eighth wonder of the world, something which doesn't seem quite accurate in your eyes. After that, you should be left in peace.

17. We've decided to have a baby. How can I be sure that my partner is the father?

From the moment you stop using contraception to the moment your pregnancy is confirmed, you must only have sexual relations with your partner. You can still be with your lovers, but steer clear of penetration. Or you could add a secondary method of contraception to the condom you usually use, such as spermicidal tampons or creams.

18. How can I ask my partner to babysit when I'm with a lover?

A baby means that you and your partner must alternate your date nights, or you will be financially ruined by babysitters! The easiest way is to decide on a specific day that each can go out. That one night a week is a welcome break in the life of a new parent, which, wonderful as it is, can be daunting, as it feels like the end of your previously carefree life. Don't feel bad about enjoying your evening, because your partner has the exact same right. As the baby gets older, the organization of your lives should become easier and easier.

19. I agree that it is important to be there for your partner when he or she needs you. But my partner only expresses this need when I have a date with someone else, as if he is trying to sabotage my other relationships or make me feel guilty. What should I do?

A need that requires your presence—such as illness, grief, or emotional distress—should not be taken lightly. But being present doesn't necessarily mean being physically at your partner's side. If he waits until you have planned a night out to express that he needs you, then he is trying to give you a guilt trip. Don't let him stop you from going out—with the exception of the serious instances mentioned above—but try to reassure him. Be gentle with him, thank him for the chance he has given you to love him in a way that's not exclusive or selfish, and explain to him that this particular outside relationship plays an important role in reinforcing your feelings toward him. Remind him that you are proud of yourself, too, for having overcome jealousy, and be happy for him in his other relationships.

20. How should we explain to our daughter that sometimes Mom and Dad go out separately?

As simply as possible: "Dad's going out with friends tonight," or "Mom's going out for dinner and you'll stay here with Dad." Young children will find this completely normal and will come to cherish the evenings where they have their mother or father all to themselves. However, if polyamory is something that you have begun later in life, after years of living in each other's pockets, then a sudden change in habits may frighten your adolescent children, who will see them as a prelude to divorce. Given that they are at the age where they are beginning to assert their independence, explain to them that now that they are older, you and your husband want to try out new things, and that it's good for you to go out without each other from time to time. Avoid talking about your specific relationships, and particularly about your sex life, just as you would avoid talking to them about theirs—unless, of course, they asked you for advice or consolation for a broken heart.

21. My son's friends saw my wife in the car with another man and told him, "Your mom is cheating on your Dad." How should I explain to him that we're not cheating on each other, but that we have a special agreement?

Tell your son that you and his mother have some friends in common, but also some that are separate—and that that's a great thing. Explain that "cheating" means lying and betraying, which neither of you is guilty of. Then make fun of his friends a little for being such gossips!

22. My lover wants to meet my children. Should I introduce her to them, and if so, how?

It's not necessary to officially involve your children in your love life by introducing them to your lover. She might want to plant ideas in their heads with not-so-subtle comments alluding to your relationship or her feelings for you. If she's not poly herself, then there's a risk she thinks in terms of emotional hierarchies and is trying to assert herself as your favorite.

If, however, you bump into your children in the street when you are out with her, or if she comes by one night to pick you up, or if she's invited to a party where your children will also be, then just introduce her as your friend, without qualifying things further. In a poly family, children know that their parents sometimes go out separately to see their own friends. An orchestrated meeting is only really necessary if you are planning to change your life around to live with your lover, which is always a possibility. Outside of this situation, though, it is advisable not to mix children with polyamory.

23. My husband is having an affair with the mother of one of our daughter's school friends. How can we avoid this kind of overlap between love life and family life?

The best way to avoid it is not to enter into these kinds of relationships. This is comparable to the traditional wisdom that advises against office romances in order to make sure that these two distinctly different universes are kept apart. The overlap already exists in your situation, so it is up to your husband and his lover to be as discreet as possible, ensuring that their respective daughters do not find out about it, as this may jeopardize their friendship.

24. One of my son's girlfriends sent me a suggestive text message. I'm flattered and tempted; what should I do?

Feeling flattered is understandable, but stay away from this temptation and from your son's terrain, where you run a high risk of hurting him. If you like younger women, there are enough on the planet to allow you to stay away from your son's friends.

25. On his way to school recently, my son wanted to come into our bedroom to say hi to me, but I had stayed overnight with a lover. My wife put him off, telling him that I was asleep and that he shouldn't wake me, but it sure was a close one! How should we deal with this in the future?

As always, the best thing to do is to tell the truth. Your wife could just as easily have said, "Dad missed the last bus and stayed overnight with friends," or, if you had gone out in the car, "Dad had a few too many drinks at dinner and decided to stay where he was rather than drive." Her response was a littler riskier and could have been problematic if your son had entered the room.

26. What should I do if a lover calls while we're eating?

One rule of etiquette, which, alas, is less and less respected these days, is that the phone should always be set to voicemail during meals, accessible only for emergency calls. If this is not the case and your lover calls, explain to her that you're eating and will call her back later. If your cell phone was on the table and you picked it up, tell your partner that it was one of your girlfriends when you hang up. Simplifying things in this way, without lies or hypocrisy, is one of polyamory's greatest merits. Frankness does not exclude discretion, however, so make sure you avoid being too lovey-dovey at the table. Of course, if your wife knows your lover, then tell her who it is so that she has a chance to say hi if she wants to.

27. How can I ask my partner to stop reading my texts and emails without it looking as though I'm hiding something from her, or that I feel guilty?

Reading other people's letters can be considered a crime, and the same should apply to modern technology. Emails are private, even if they are not love letters. Given the general independence within poly relationships, each partner will have their own email address and cell phone. If your partner refuses to stop reading your messages, create a password that is too hard for her to guess (i.e., not your date of birth), and remind her that going through a man's pockets won't stop him from running away—and might instead give him the impression that he is under surveillance. However, your comment about feeling guilty makes me wonder if you have accepted that you have a right to a private life to which she does not have access. This is something that you should really think about.

28. I called my lover five times without getting through. He saw the missed calls and accused me of stalking him. How can I make him understand that I was just trying to call him, and that not a single possessive thought even crossed my mind?

You don't have to explain anything. If he feels harassed, that signifies that he is insecure in the relationship, or that he is trying to destabilize you with this "proof" of your jealous and possessive nature. Trying to justify your actions will only confirm his convictions. Stop calling him for a while; let some time go by. If he doesn't call back, then the first theory was probably correct: he didn't feel good within the relationship. If it's hard for you not to call him, then perhaps he was right about the second theory. A poly woman is as susceptible as anyone to fall head over heels in love, and can experience the same feelings of fragility and anxiety. It's a big mistake to deny that by pretending to be tough all the time.

29. I always block caller ID from my phone to keep my number private. Unfortunately, one of my lovers never

answers the call if it comes up as restricted. What should I do?

I'm no pro when it comes to cell phone technology, but I think that you can arrange things so that his phone rings in a special tone when you call, without displaying your number. You could also agree on a code: let it ring twice, hang up, then call again. That way he'll know it's you.

30. How should I protect myself against sexually transmitted diseases (STDs), and with which partners?

Polyamory comes hand-in-hand with condom use. This method protects against HIV and many other STDs, though not all. Fortunately, with the exception of AIDS, the majority of these are treatable with effective modern medicine. In theory, you should use protection with all lovers in any instances where bodily fluids are exchanged. This includes your long-term partner if you can't be sure of how careful he or she is being with others. In practice, most poly men and women decide to use protection at all times except with their life partner. Others form "safe-sex communities" by only choosing lovers who are regularly tested for HIV. Still others, basing their information on epidemiological research concerning sexual practices, only use a condom if they consider their risk factor to be statistically significant.

31. When should I bring up the condom issue?

As soon as you broach the fact that you are "faithful but not exclusive." Point out that the only downside to this lifestyle choice is that it means condoms are obligatory. And make sure you always have one with you.

32. I picked up a sexually transmitted disease that is benign but contagious. Should I warn everyone I have sex with from now on?

In the case of contagious STDs, it is very important that you inform all of your sexual partners, so that they can get treatment and not pass it on any further. Remember that some STDs are more easily cured for men but can cause sterility or cervical cancer for women if they are not detected and treated in time. Given that trust is such an important part of polyamory, it goes without saying that anyone who is HIV positive should tell their future lovers at the very beginning, even if they always use condoms.

33. I'm single and usually bring my lovers back to my place. Should I change the sheets each time?

Speaking on both a hygienic and symbolic level, it is certainly preferable. Of course, this becomes quite a job if you have a different partner every night, but things rarely happen at quite such a frenetic rate with polyamory. Also, there's nothing to stop you from going to a hotel every now and then to avoid these chores, or from choosing a designated spot for each of your partners in your apartment: the bed, the living room couch, the office rug, and so on.

34. How can I be sure I'm not getting involved with a psychopath?

It is hard to tell if someone is psychotic before they reach their breaking point. Fortunately, such mental illness only affects about 2 percent of the population, a figure that is roughly the same around the world, and even within that 2 percent, few are dangerous. Whether you are poly or not, your chances of meeting a criminal pervert are pretty slim. However, there are certain things that you can do to create a safer environment and to test out whether your date is "normal" or not. The large majority of rapists are not psychopaths in the medical sense of the term, but are rather men who give in suddenly to impulses that they have been repressing.

To avoid walking into a dangerous situation, make sure your first few dates with a new prospective lover are in public places. Try to get as much information about him as possible: who he is, what he does, where he works, and so forth. He will be happy that you're so interested in him, and you will have a better chance of sussing him out. Take his phone number, but don't give him yours; it's true that this puts you in the position of making the next move, but it also prevents him from finding out where you live before you're ready to tell him. Don't go to his place right away, and if you do, make sure to give his address to a friend, and arrange for her to call you in an hour, letting him know that you are expecting a call. Warn your partner if you plan to stay out overnight, so that he will know something is wrong if you don't come home when he was expecting you. If you go home with someone you don't know well, make sure you leave your phone on, as this will allow the police to trace you if need be.

Remember that poly women are not at any higher risk than other women of getting into a dangerous situation. In fact, the opposite is often true, thanks to poly women's extensive knowledge of men, their ability to identify odd behavior, and their tendency to not let passion run away with them.

35. Dating several women gets expensive, especially if I'm a "gentleman" and pay for everything. Can I suggest that we split the check without looking like a cheapskate?

It's the not the number of women that becomes pricey, but the number of dates. If you eat out at a restaurant with your wife every night, you'll spend as much as you would if you went on dates with seven different women in one week! In any case, the man paying is a custom that is on its way out, especially for poly women, who feel particularly strongly about gender equality. However, breaking out the calculator at the end of a meal to divide up the check is a bit of a turn-off. It is more exciting to take turns picking up the check. This ritual could be the prelude to an erotic game, where the one who pays becomes the master/mistress of the rest of the evening in a classic fantasy of "buying what you want." Or perhaps the lover who cooked dinner then offers himself to the other: "Do what you want to me, I am your dessert!"

36. I like to get dressed up for a night out, but I love relaxing in jeans and running shoes at home. How can I make sure that my husband doesn't feel like I treat the other men in my life better than him?

The same goes for your partner: if he falls asleep in his sweats in front of the TV with you, but you see him all spruced up to go out on a date, you will quickly lose desire for him. This is one of the difficulties of polyamory.

Love means that you can reveal your true self to your partner, and be accepted and cherished even when you are tired, sick, or in a bad mood. Over the years, this level of intimacy will create a bond that is much stronger than that of seduction, but you must make sure that the latter does not disappear completely. Your partner will understandably feel frustrated if it seems that the two of you only share serious things—passionate as they may sometimes be—and that you save your playful self for your lovers. If you don't feel like dressing up in sexy lingerie and high heels for him, then remind him with a smile just how lucky he is to see you in your athletic wear—something that none of your lovers has ever seen. You can even incorporate your outfit into an erotic game: let yourself be inspired by those advertisements for tight-fitting jeans, the top button undone for a sexy pose. And the games don't have to be all about sex: you could leave secret notes for each other, exchange sensual massages, or go on impromptu little adventures. The important thing is to share the pleasure of playfulness and to enjoy being carefree together.

37. What should I do with the love letters I receive?

Love letters on paper are rare these days, and therefore precious. They are a moving testament to the past when we read them years later, helping us remember the incredible moments we experienced. Letters also help keep the spirit of lost lovers alive. Keeping them or throwing them away is dictated by the relationship you have with the past. If you decide to keep them, be sure to file them away in an envelope marked "confidential."

Your children or grandchildren may wish to read them one day down the line, but at least they will have had prior warning that they are entering a private universe, and that they do so at their own risk. You could also specify "to be destroyed on my death" as a last wish.

Testimonials

The following testimonials do not paint the picture of polyamory as if it were a lifestyle choice that is constantly bathed in light. They outline the difficulties that this choice can give rise to, which must be dealt with by the individuals concerned, given that the rest of society is just waiting to see them fail. Life in the poly world has its ups and downs just like anywhere else, but the following extracts show how fulfilling a compliment such a life can be for those with intelligent, sensual, radiant personalities.

E wrote to me for the first time in January 2003, and we have been corresponding ever since. We have met twice, and I include a few extracts from her letters:

I am forty years old, and after seeing you on TV a few weeks ago, I am dying to get to know you. You were talking about your life and I recognized myself. It made me so happy to see that other women see life as I do and are not afraid to say so. For a long time now I have felt quite alone. I am married to a wonderful man, but I think that my desire scares him. I love my husband, but I don't want to give up my sexuality. Three years ago, on vacation, I met another man, who was so kind and took a real interest in me. We had coffee together in the afternoon, and the next evening I accepted his invitation to have a drink at his place. I knew what was going to happen . . . and it was wonderful. It could have just been a holiday romance, but it ended up blossoming into something quite beautiful. We fell in love. We see each other once or twice a year now, and each time we spend just a few days together—what wonderful, carefree, sensual days! I love my husband, but I am in love with my lover. I need them both.

June 2003

I recently had a very disappointing experience with a man who completely mistook me for some sort of glutton, just out for what I could get. To make myself feel better, I reread your letter and To Love Several Men. *I feel quite isolated at the moment and feel that my husband is the only one who truly understands my beliefs and my life-view! I am so lucky to have such an understanding husband, and his acceptance of me only makes me love him more. . . .*

July 2003

I am a middle-aged woman and I feel like I am only now beginning to understand the joys of male company! I'm currently reading your novel, Latitudes of Love. *On days when my soul feels like a rainy November sky, your words shine down like rays of sunshine.*

. . . You seem to bring me good luck: I have just met a very special man. His intelligence, his sensitivity, his voice . . . I go weak at the knees. I want to thank you for the doors you have opened in my life.

December 2003

My little garden of men is finally coming into bloom. All I need is two or three more rare species to brighten up the beds . . .

In 2004, E met several wonderful men, but also a few disappointing ones. In 2005, she met a "delicious epicurean" with whom she shared some particularly beautiful times, but she then decided to take a break from her love life to dedicate more time to the theater, a field she wished to throw herself into further. The following year was a quiet one, because her husband was having some serious work issues and needed her at his side.

Letter from C, thirty-six years old:

February 2008

I read your book with great satisfaction: I finally realize that I'm not an alien after all! This love for other people has been growing inside of me for some time now, held back by my upbringing, by society, by my family . . . and for a long time, by myself. I dabbled a little, but my inability to fully accept it stopped me from being able to enjoy it. Today, however, at thirty-six, I live my romances to the max, falling in love in almost every instance (to my despair!), but with a greater ability to bounce back each time! This has been my view on life for as long as I've been married, but I just didn't know how to go about loving more than one man. As soon as I picked up your book, it felt as if my prayers had been answered, and I savored every page.

P, forty-seven, is a friend I have often talked to about polyamory. He is so discreet about his private life that I had always assumed that he was pretty much monogamous. But he knew that I was on the lookout for testimonials for this book, so he sent me this letter:

October 2008

There are three women in my life at the moment. One is an artist, one in academia, and the other does manual work. My work doesn't allow for much free time, and they are all fairly demanding, but I can see that it excites them that I am hard to pin down. I love all three dearly, but I couldn't live with any of them because I need to have time to myself. I have no desire to live as part of a couple and don't understand the necessity. The thing I love is getting to know their different personalities, in life and in the bedroom. I don't usually talk to my lovers about polyamory immediately. Nor do I avoid their questions, but I find that they don't usually ask many. However, I'm sure that they can tell from my erotic tastes and my insistence on using condoms that they are not the only ones in my life.

For me, a relationship is only really complete when there is sexual intimacy. I have three very close guy friends and am straight, so I feel that, having no sexual attraction to them, there will always be a part of them, this secret dimension, that I will never know. Sex is what allows you to really get inside someone's head, to come face-to-face with the most mysterious part of their being. That's what I love so much. I am fortunate to be living the wonderful things that I am. The only bad thing is that with lovers who are looking to become part of a couple, breakup is often inevitable.

B was in the audience for a television show I was a guest on. After the show, she asked if we could meet, and we have now been corresponding regularly since 2004, during which period we have met several times:

July 2004

Dear Françoise, we are going to change the romantic world as we know it, but it's going to take a little time. As for us, there's not a minute to be lost; we are so lucky to be alive and must make the most of it! As time goes on, I meet more and more men and women who think like us and who are breaking down boundaries, leaving guilt in the dust. Life, friendships, feelings, sex . . . these pleasures should be celebrated! Let's not complicate things unnecessarily. As for me, I'm leaving work and am off to catch the train to meet my darling

T___. My head is already spinning. Women like us are the future for men! When will the media turn its attentions to relationships that function perfectly well without this rigid fidelity? Isn't true love stronger than sexual exclusivity?

July 2005

As I said briefly on the phone, I'm a bit out of it at the moment, as changes at work are taking up most of my time. Because of these ups and downs, I'm going through a bit of a dry patch, romance-wise. My libido is low at the moment for the first time in my life. I don't feel like myself at all. At least I realize that this is probably just temporary and that I'll be back on track soon. My husband isn't ready to leave his job, so I'll be up here on my placement without him. Perhaps this is the perfect time for him to embrace the independence he has so far been reluctant even to imagine? Maybe this new sense of autonomy will lead him into the arms of a mistress? I really do hope so. . . .

September 2008, with a broken heart

I have learned that life is easier for women when they think like men! What attraction is there for a man in a woman who has decided to live in the moment? Most of the men I meet prefer to obsessively analyze the character of the woman they would like to seduce, to try to figure out how they can be sure that what seems like a great opportunity isn't going to turn into a nightmare. "Is this ravishing woman, teetering on the edge of hysteria, going to disrupt my tidy little life and tear me apart? Or is she going to become a sumptuous lover and friend?" What a dilemma, the poor things!

It's official: men are from Mars and women are from Venus! I believe that only when we understand that men simply aren't programmed to think in the same way as us, can we really say that we are FREE! The moment that I understood that I had been brought up to think like a woman and that it wasn't working for me, I decided to start thinking like a man, and found that I felt much more comfortable! In fact, that was the moment that I feel like I really became myself!

It was just after seeing you on TV, on the show where someone was accusing you of "stealing husbands" (you are such a threat to married women!). You explained that you weren't stealing anything, but that you simply borrowed them and returned them in the same, if not better, condition! The ease with which you spoke opened my eyes to just how much my own way of thinking—pre-programmed and boxed in—was completely backward! I finally saw that the anxiety that was keeping me down was a direct consequence of my efforts to be something that I'm not. I had been living for too long in someone else's skin, and I decided it was time for a change. I took a different look at my life and realized that I liked what I saw. I stopped seeing men as "husbands" or "pigs." I banished the years' worth of clichés and preconceptions that were holding me back and finally confronted my true desires, welcomed my fantasies onboard, and reinstated pleasure to its rightful place at the top of my priorities. Thanks to you, my life started over again, albeit tentatively at the beginning. I couldn't help be-

ing hesitant at first, but bit by bit my confidence grew and I came to accept that I wasn't stealing anybody's husband either. I discovered that it was possible to love more than one man in more than one way without encroaching on their lives or my own. In fact, quite the opposite, the new experiences and emotions only enhanced the lives of everyone involved. Since I began this new life (my real life!), I have been extraordinarily lucky: I have only met wonderful men, luscious lovers. I've never had a bad date or an unpleasant surprise, only happiness. Each has a place in my heart, and I have never suffered any argument or misunderstanding. With any one of them, I could pick up the phone tomorrow and it would be as if we had only just hung up yesterday, even if it had in fact been six months since we had had any contact. I call these men my special friends. There are some who have not been lovers for years but they could quite easily become such tomorrow if the occasion presented itself.

This lifestyle is harder to lead out here in the country, which is why most of my lovers are in Paris. Not that the moral atmosphere is necessarily more restrictive in the country, but it is more difficult on a practical level. You find yourself looking over your shoulder, afraid of being seen or running into the wrong person at the wrong moment. Paris offers delicious afternoons of mischief and wild nights . . . for no man is the same under the covers. To the women who say that all men make love in the same way, I say, "No! They're all different!" They all have slightly different techniques, and that's what makes polyamory so much fun!

I have never had a special friend that hurt me or made me suffer in any way, and I love them for that too. We're here for pleasure, not pain, and for years that is how it has been for me, with every single one of them.

So then why, with X, has everything gone so wrong? I shouldn't have let myself get in so deep. I thought I was immune to disappointment and let myself get carried away with my feelings for him. There seemed to be only one way to go: straight ahead! But then I suddenly realized that while I was going straight ahead . . . I was doing so alone. He didn't want to be just "special friends." He said that it was not enough for us, but, at the same time, he wouldn't go so far as to join me on the road to love, which he must have seen as a dangerous one for him. X is probably the only man I've ever met who didn't know where things were going with me. All the others know, just as I know where I'm going with them. That's why things are so uncomplicated and easily sustainable. But with X, things got complicated too quickly. I knew where I was going but he didn't, despite his insistence to the contrary, and that is what ruined our beautiful romance.

M. C., thirty-one years old, referenced one of my books on the swingers blog that she and her husband, G., write. I have met them both on several occasions:

August 2008
My husband is a real Don Juan, who just loves to flirt, and I knew when we married that he would not be faithful. For ten years the conversation just never

came up. About three years into our marriage, I had an affair, which I kept secret. Then after ten years I accidently discovered—his email gave him away—that G. had a mistress. I confronted him, and he gave me the classic male retort: "It was just one night!" However, he was surprised by how tolerant I was. We discussed it at length, I confessed to my previous affair, and we decided to give swinging a go. Now we enjoy erotic parties in clubs and also have lovers outside of our relationship, the details of which I prefer to keep to myself. He likes to tell me about his, but I need my little secret garden!

This freedom has so many advantages: I don't feel guilty or compelled to lie, I can move about freely without inventing excuses to go out, I'm actually turned on by the fear of my husband falling in love somewhere else, and the fact that our relationship is so unconventional has only brought us closer together. There are drawbacks, of course: if nothing is forbidden, then we risk letting our open relationship fall into a pattern. Perhaps we'll get bored with our sexual adventures and will have to "increase the dose" or push the boundaries even further in order to maintain the level of desire. Keeping our lifestyle a secret from our child, from our families, and from most of our friends can be exhausting sometimes, but we're not sure how to bring it up with them, or if we should even bother.

We trust each other so much that I never feel jealous. I think I probably would if he gave me all the raunchy details of his nights out. Strangely, though, I have experienced some feelings of jealousy toward the wife of one of my lovers!

Of our thirteen years of marriage, we've only been living in this way for three, so it is too early to really assess the impact it has had. We just take things one step at a time, discussing it as we go . . . almost too much sometimes. When I feel that our love life is dominating our conversations, I sometimes worry that we are obsessed with it, to the detriment of the other things we like to do.

Letter from F:

January 2004

It gave me great pleasure to read your distinction between "faithful" and "exclusive" in To Love Several Men, *something which I have been trying to explain to people for ten years now. I have even dedicated several pages of writing to it myself, trying to differentiate between these two notions, a differentiation that the large majority of women seems to be fundamentally, culturally unprepared to accept. If my experience is anything to go by, then I must tell you that your way of thinking is rare in a woman. And those men who share it rarely dare to talk about it. As for me, my friends and family think of me as a swinger, as someone strange (they call it polyfidelity!), but they also understand that I'm a serious, thoughtful person.*

Letter from J. Y.:

August 2003

I have been living the life that you describe for the last twenty years, since my divorce. My newfound freedom has taught me that I am a faithful person: I find it hard to leave people. That's how, twenty years on, I find myself surrounded by girlfriends at the age of sixty-five! I see some of them often, some very rarely, but I continue to feel a strong connection to each. I see one of these women just once a year and can't describe the happiness I feel as the date gets closer—the emotional reunion, the sadness when we say goodbye, always wondering how things will be next year. Then, in a more general sense, there's the excitement of taking a train to meet a girlfriend in the country or overseas. But, as you point out, things are not always this easy. The problem for men, particularly single men, is to make women understand the concept of non-exclusivity. Reading your words gave me hope, not just because of the arguments you develop, but because of their fundamental roots: the kindness and love of mankind.

An email from S:

August 2008

Love, for me, comes in all the colors of the rainbow. I don't collect "trophies," like a huntress or a warrior, and I have no bones to pick with the so-called "stronger" sex. I just take care of each color of love that enters my life. To my future ex-husband, I offer the capital L of Love, branded by passion, and solid as a rock. Fifteen years of extraordinary joy, but also pain. Circumstance dictates that we go our separate ways, but he'll always be the king of my life and, in some ways, I wish for no other husband, no other relationship, no other name than his.

*Then there's my artist-lover, one of life's great
rebels, for whom my love comes in fits and starts. I lose
myself in the whirlwind of ever-changing games, surprises, emotions, and still find that there is room for
deep feelings to evolve. I love, too, the fragile, secretive,
mature man who recently entered my life. A few years
ago, I went wild for the lover who unleashed my inner
animal, but I love with an intense, asexual affection
the man, twenty-four years my senior, who over time
has become my best friend, my soul mate, my confidant.
I won't list them all here, but those I care for, each in a
unique manner, know the place that they occupy in my
heart, just as I know those who hold me dear. I yearn
for the natural harmony that is born from simplicity,
not a relationship that requires work and sacrifice. So I
let things come (or not) at their own speed, and let time
take care of time. I want to be free to enjoy an afternoon
or night with a loved one (sex or no sex) without having
to deal with another's long face the next day, without
him worrying that the place he holds in my heart is in
danger. I lay claim to my "private garden"—or, as my
husband maliciously called it, my "vegetable garden."
This right should be a given in any relationship, but
still needs to be demanded—it is as important to me as
the air that I breathe. Likewise the ability to form close
ties with lovers, and I allow the men I hold close to have
access to both.*

L. S., whose internet pseudonym is "Long Legs," contacted me through my blog, and we met up one weekend
in the town where she lives. Also present were V., the

author of the opening letter of this book, and S., another wonderful poly woman. It was a surprising weekend of sweetness and harmony. Long Legs' lover, James, was also there and was blown away by our opinions, which were so far removed from those common in his own culture. Several months later, L. S. and James separated because they were unable to bridge the gap between their different worlds.

L. S. wrote this piece, which sums up perfectly the concept of polyamory:

> *James is my type of guy. But I don't want to give up the others, the next, the previous, the new.*
>
> *That doesn't necessarily mean that they'll be sexual relationships. There are no rules: just desire, yearning, and tenderness, the conductors of love. I want to share the intellectual discoveries I make with James, to share the things I learn from my friends, male and female. I don't want him to worry when I give my hand to, or fall into the arms of, those who move me. James knows this; I told him in a letter. His views are different, and I accept that. I'm not currently attracted to anybody else sexually, but I won't say "never," that's all. People think that by not saying "never," you want to jump on the next person hwo arouses even the slightest desire in you. But it's more subtle, more special, deeper than that. Right now, if a man invited me into his arms, I couldn't do it, no matter how perfect, how funny, how seductive he might be. I am too caught up with James.*
>
> *I am going to lose him because he won't accept polyamory. But if I agree to be exclusive with him, I will lose*

my other lovers. I know deep down that I will always love him as much as I do now, regardless of distance, silence, separation. That's what I don't want to lose: the love I feel for him. Just as I have never lost that feeling with the others. When I see them again, it's real, it's pure bliss, just as it was with Génie the other day. He and I don't sleep together, but the charm, the intimate feelings, the complicity of our conversations are there because we both know that if we so desired, we would make love like two adults, free in our choices.

Several weeks later, Long Legs and James met up again, discussed things and got together:

I feel that a weight has been lifted off my shoulders again. I am through with allowing my freedom to love—who and when I want—to be boxed in by an obligation to fidelity. James and I meet for a drink, or at his place, or at mine if the kids are out, and we make love with love. Our discussions are deep and serious without being dark. I love it. Pascal writes to me as well. I write back, often with tears in my eyes. We still need to confide in each other, to tell the other, "I still love you." So we lunch together with the children, who are happy to see him and his kids again. Sometimes we go to a gallery and laugh, like the old days. He has a sweet, gentle lover now, but he says I'm still the woman of his life. It's a shame he didn't realize that a little earlier. I see him in a different light now, not the light of love, but filtered nonetheless through the heart that has always loved him. But I'm in love with James.

*And then there's William, whom I get on so well
with and could listen to all day. He confides in me, tells
me about his heartbreaks, his need to be free, the gentle-
manly impulse that leads him to spoil his ex-lover's kids.
Willaim treats me like his sister, like his best friend, like
the person he can ask anything of, safe in the knowledge
that she'll have no qualms saying no.*

*And then sometimes Génie pops up. My nights with
him are pure delight! His subtle, light soul and sense
of humor never fail to raise my spirits. When we walk
together, arm in arm, I feel like a child, free and happy.*

*That's where my life is at right now. I'm also draw-
ing and painting more! And living the single life, in
love with James, happy in the knowledge that if I want
to embrace one of my loves, with a kiss or something
more, then I will. Life is good.*

Letter from Professor C. H.:

August 2005
This summer I read To Love Several Men. *I am
an anthropologist and a doctor working in the field of
exclusion and violence. For twenty years now I have
been involved in violence-prevention programs, and I
was extremely impressed by the ideas you brought up
and developed. Your perception of sexuality is true to
life, and the openness you propose is a feasible way to
improve relations between men and women in the realm
of love, which, instead of bringing them closer together,
is too often a pretext for hatred.*

Never Forever, Never Never . . .

When *To Love Several Men* came out in 2002, I expected to arouse the curiosity and skepticism of journalists, and I was not disappointed! I was also hoping for the opportunity to compare my experiences with those of other poly men and women, and a few did come forward. But only a few, for the majority of the "open" relationships that started in the 1970s did not end up making it.

On the other hand, and this was a welcome surprise, I heard from many men and women who had not previously been able to put their finger on the anxiety their relationships were causing them. These were relationships they had both aspired to and dreaded, and they were relieved now to discover that there were other possible ways of living, free from dogma and in accordance with life's cycles. I had cleared a path which, these days, is increasingly trodden by men and women, particularly young people looking to avoid repeating the pattern of serial monogamy—marriage, divorce, marriage, divorce—that affected the lives of many of them as children. Websites such as *www.polyamorysociety.org* and *www .worldpolyamoryassociation.org* have become venues for high-level discussions of a moral and philosophical nature, which show that younger generations are seeking a life that has direction, that is coherent, and that offers attention to the other in such a way that it makes the future seem optimistic, even if there is still a long way to go.[29]

I will let my life partner, the father of my daughters, have the last word here. He told me one day, "You have taught me that we should never say 'never' and never say 'forever' when it comes to love. That everything is possible." And also, "I have never deprived myself of a single thing under the pretext that we are married."

I cannot think of a better way to summarize the joy of polyamory.

---

29 Translator's note: the French-language websites originally referenced were *www.polyamour.info*, *www.polyamour.be*, and *www.iledessens.com*.

Bibliography

Robin Baker, *Sperm Wars:Infidelity, Sexual Conflict and Other Bedroom Battles*

Philippe Brenot, *Inventer le couple*

Sophie Cadalen, *Les autres*

Françoise Chandernagor, *La première épouse*

Serge Chaumier, *L'amour fissionnel*

John Gray, *Men are from Mars, Women are from Venus*

Benoîte Groult, *Les vaisseaux du coeur*

Serge Hefez and Danièle Laufer, *La danse du couple*

Dzongsar Jamyang Khyentse, *What Makes You Not a Buddhist*

Henri Laborit, *In Praise of Fleeing*

Aldo Naouri, *Adultères*

Willy Pasini, *Éloge de l'intimité*

Mazarine Pingeot, *Bouche cousue*

Wilhelm Reich, *The Sexual Revolution*

Paule Salomon, *Bienheureuse infidélité*

Jean-Didier Vincent, *The Biology of Emotions*

Lucy Vincent, *Comment devient-on amoureux?*